Powered Endoscopic Sinus Surgery

Powered Endoscopic Sinus Surgery

John H. Krouse, M.D., Ph.D., F.A.C.S.
Florida Sinus Center
Ormond Beach, Florida

Dewey A. Christmas, Jr., M.D.
Florida Sinus Center
Ormond Beach, Florida

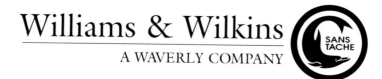

Williams & Wilkins
A WAVERLY COMPANY

BALTIMORE • PHILADELPHIA • LONDON • PARIS • BANGKOK
BUENOS AIRES • HONG KONG • MUNICH • SYDNEY • TOKYO • WROCLAW

Editor: Darlene Barela Cooke
Managing Editor: Frances M. Klass
Production Coordinator: Dana M. Soares
Typesetter: Better Graphics, Inc.
Printer: Quebecor Printing

Copyright © 1997 Williams & Wilkins

351 West Camden Street
Baltimore, Maryland 21201–2436 USA

Rose Tree Corporate Center
1400 North Providence Road
Building II, Suite 5025
Media, Pennsylvania 19063–2043 USA

Accurate indications, adverse reactions and dosage schedules for drugs are provided in this book, but it is possible that they may change. The reader is urged to review the package information data of the manufacturers of the medications mentioned.

Printed in the United States of America

First Edition,

ISBN: 0-683-30351-1

The publishers have made every effort to trace the copyright holders for borrowed material. If they have inadvertently overlooked any, they will be pleased to make the necessary arrangements at the first opportunity.

To purchase additional copies of this book, call our customer service department at **(800) 638-0672** or fax orders to **(800) 447-8438.** For other book services, including chapter reprints and large quantity sales, ask for the Special Sales department.

Canadian customers should call **(800) 665-1148,** or fax **(800) 665-0103.** For all other calls originating outside of the United States, please call **(410) 528-4223** or fax us at **(410) 528-8550.**

Visit *Williams & Wilkins* on the Internet: http://www.wwilkins.com or contact our customer service department at **custserv@wwilkins.com.** Williams & Wilkins customer service representatives are available from 8:30 am to 6:00 pm, EST, Monday through Friday, for telephone access.

97 98 99 00
1 2 3 4 5 6 7 8 9 10

Forward

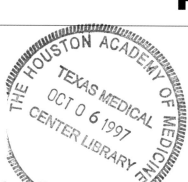

Powered instrumentation has dramatically improved our ability to deal with patients who present with massive polyposis. Microdebrider technology delivers many of the advantages that we had hoped to achieve with laser surgery, at less cost and with less scarring.

The authors have put together a detailed book, which clearly delineates the potential use of microdebriders for polypectomy, as well as separate chapters detailing their potential use in each of the sinuses. The authors are to be particularly congratulated for the sections on surgical and radiographic anatomy. The section on surgical anatomy by Eiji Yanigasawa is precise and as richly illustrated as one would expect from this author who is such an outstanding endoscopic photographer. It appears to

be well augmented by the radiographic anatomy and radiographic images of Ramon Figueroa. In addition to the detailed sections covering the use of a microdebrider in each of the sinuses, such issues as dacryocystorhinostomy, complications and future directions are also covered.

In addition to a careful review of the anatomy, this book therefore carefully details many of the current techniques for the use of powered instrumentation in sinus surgery. It provides worthwhile information for otolaryngologists embarking on the use of powered instrumentation in their practice.

David W. Kennedy, M.D.
Chairperson, Department of Otolaryngology
University of Pennsylvania.

Acknowledgements

We wish to thank Dr. Eiji Yanagisawa for his unwavering encouragement, friendship, and support.

We also wish to thank Dr. David Kennedy for introducing us to functional endoscopic sinus surgery, for being a friend and mentor, and for his gracious writing of the foreword to this textbook.

We further wish to acknowledge Dr. Gerald Wolf for encouraging us to pursue the use of powered technology in sinus surgery, which has permitted the development of these exciting new methods.

We also wish to thank Rick Purcell, Dennis Kennedy, and Caroline Parker for their expertise and assistance in the operating room which has allowed us to adopt these techniques and document our work through photography.

And, finally, we would like to thank our wives, Helene and Sandra, for their love, encouragement, and support throughout the often tedious and time-consuming process of authoring this text.

J.H.K.
D.A.C.

Preface

In June 1993 one of us (D.A.C.) had the pleasure of hosting Dr. Gery Wolf from Graz, Austria on his family's visit to Florida. At a dinner in Orlando, Dr. Wolf asked if we had tried a special vacuum rotary dissection device used by orthopedic surgeons for any of our sinus surgery procedures. While we had not considered such an idea prior to this dinner, the concept was quite intriguing. On returning home to Daytona Beach, we asked one of the circulating nurses if she had experience with this instrument. Much to our delight she retrieved a long-discarded powered dissection device which had been abandoned by the oral surgeons after their interest in temporomandibular joint surgery had waned.

We began using this device in our sinus surgical cases shortly after Dr. Wolf's visit. At first, we tried using the instrument on one side, while performing surgery on the contralateral side using standard techniques. It became clear very quickly that the sinuses dissected with the powered debrider were healing more rapidly than with the standard procedure, with less bleeding and with excellent results. We soon adopted powered surgery of the sinuses as our primary method for all of our cases. The powered revolution was underway!

It is clear that the evolution and expansion of powered techniques in functional endoscopic sinus surgery have been among the most exciting developments of the decade in otolaryngology. The number of sinus surgeons who are adopting these methods is increasing exponentially, and the scientific literature supporting powered surgical techniques is growing. Despite the recent interest in powered endoscopic sinus surgery, no textbook has yet examined this area. The present text has been designed for that purpose—to provide a thorough description of powered techniques in functional endoscopic sinus surgery for the practicing otolaryngologist. In our opinion these techniques represent a significant advance in the surgical treatment of sinus disease. We are pleased to offer this textbook to the otolaryngology community.

John H. Krouse, M.D., Ph.D., F.A.C.S.
Dewey A. Christmas, Jr., M.D.
Ormond Beach, Florida

Contributors

Dewey A. Christmas, Jr., M.D.
Florida Sinus Center
Ormond Beach, Florida

Ramón E. Figueroa, M.D.
Associate Professor of Radiology and
    Chief, Section of Neuroradiology
Medical College of Georgia
Augusta, Georgia

Helene J. Krouse, Ph.D., R.N., C.S., A.R.N.P.
Associate Professor and Acting Chairperson
Department of Nursing
College of Health
University of North Florida
Jacksonville, Florida

John H. Krouse, M.D., Ph.D., F.A.C.S.
Florida Sinus Center
Ormond Beach, Florida

Michael A. Mercandetti, M.D.
Private Practice
Huntington, New York

Joseph P. Mirante, M.D., M.B.A., F.A.C.S.
Florida Sinus Center
Ormond Beach, Florida

B. Manrin Rains III, M.D., F.A.C.S.
Director, Mid-South Sinus Center
Memphis, Tennessee

James Stankiewicz, M.D., F.A.C.S.
Department of Otolaryngology–Head and Neck
    Surgery
Loyola University Medical Center
Maywood, Illinois

Eiji Yanagisawa, M.D., F.A.C.S.
Clinical Professor of Otolaryngology
Yale University School of Medicine
Attending Otolaryngologist, Hospital of St. Raphael
New Haven, Connecticut

Contents

Introduction to Powered Technology in Otolaryngology

John H. Krouse, M.D., Ph.D., F.A.C.S.
Dewey A. Christmas, Jr., M.D.

By all accounts, the rapid growth in the use of powered instrumentation in functional endoscopic sinus surgery has been a revolution in the current practice of otolaryngology. Since the first implementation of this technology for sinus surgery in 1992 through the present time, the use of various power-driven devices has attracted many supporters due to its improved safety and precision and through its ease of use. The proliferation of dissection courses throughout the country and the increased exposure given the technology at national and regional meetings further demonstrate the growing popularity of this method.

HISTORY

The concept of a power-driven, suction-based rotating surgical system was first developed by Dr. Jack Urban of the House Ear Institute in the late 1960s. The device was designed for use in the removal of acoustic neuromas, and was patented by Dr. Urban on March 6, 1969 (Vacuum Rotary Dissector, Figure 1.1).[1] The original model is still in use at the House Ear Institute in neuro-otologic procedures (personal communication, John House, October 1, 1996). Since that time, various types of soft tissue shavers and rotary dissectors have been in broad use in orthopedics for arthroscopic surgery. In addition, smaller versions of these devices were employed by oral surgeons in the 1980s for arthroscopic surgery

of the temporomandibular joint (TMJ). As these procedures have become somewhat less common, many of the early sinus surgical cases using powered instrumentation were completed using abandoned TMJ devices. With the increasing popularity of powered surgery of the sinuses, various manufacturers have developed instrumentation specifically for use in these procedures.

The first report of the use of powered instrumentation in functional endoscopic sinus surgery was by Setliff and Parsons[2] in 1994. The authors reported on their experience with 345 patients ranging in age from 3 to 85 years. They used a powered device generically referred to as a "microdebrider," a rotating shaver which drew tissue into an inner cannula and sharply sheared it off. This device was referred to as the Hummer™ (Stryker Corporation, Santa Clara, CA) due to the manner in which the device "hummed" through the tissue. Setliff has continued to popularize the technique through dissection courses and instruction of otolaryngologists in the technique, and has been one of its major advocates since its introduction.

The microdebriders were first marketed to otolaryngologists for soft tissue work, and have been widely described as devices for the removal of polypoid tissue in the nose and sinuses. Hawke and McCombe[3] describe their experience in the removal of nasal polyps in the office setting. In their series of 50 patients, the authors note that removal of tissue was quite easy, with minimal bleeding. Hawke and

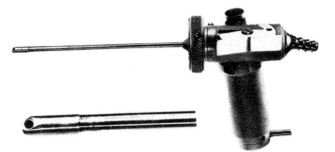

Fig. 1.1 Urban Vacuum Rotary Dissector, 1968 (reprinted with permission).

McCombe found that nasal packing was unnecessary due to the precise removal of tissue with the microdebrider. Similar findings were reported by Krouse and Christmas,[4] in a report of 35 patients who underwent office nasal polypectomy using the microdebrider. In this study bleeding was minimal and nasal packing was not necessary. Again the precision of the device was noted, and its ability to remove tissue with minimal secondary trauma was described.

Christmas and Krouse[5] reported their technique in powered dissection of the paranasal sinuses in 1996. In this article, the authors described their specific method to total sphenoethmoidectomy in a sequential manner, noting again the increased precision and safety of the technique. The majority of surgeons who utilize powered technology continue to do so in major part for dissection of polypoid tissue, and then revert to traditional techniques for the bulk of the sinus work. Krouse and Christmas, however, noted their experience with extensive bony work of the sinuses using this device. They described their experience with their first 250 patients who underwent powered surgery of the sinuses.[6] They noted decreased intraoperative bleeding, faster healing times, less postoperative scarring and synechia formation, and equivalent symptom relief in the powered dissection group. The authors attributed these findings to decreased trauma to normal tissue, less deepithelialization of bone, and the seaming action of the device as tissue is sheared free. Krouse and Christmas clearly demonstrate that powered dissection is not a technique which is limited to soft tissue work alone.

Gross and Becker[7] also have written on the use of microdebriders in their practice of endoscopic sinus surgery. They report that the use of this technology allows a clearer surgical field during surgery, with particular utility in cases of severe polyposis and in revision surgery. They confirm that stripping of normal mucosa seems to be decreased through the use of these devices, and that results of the surgery using these devices are comparable to that seen with traditional surgical techniques.

With the easy removal of polypoid tissue from the nose and sinuses, manufacturers have begun to introduce various brands and models of microdebriders to the marketplace. These devices are all effective in the removal of soft tissue and polypoid disease. The field of sinus surgery, however, has begun to move more toward the completion of the entire sphenoethmoidectomy with a powered device alone. It has become apparent that most of the powered instruments available for sale do not have the requisite power to remove the bony partitions in the ethmoid labyrinth or to enlarge the bony borders of the maxillary ostium. As a result, all of the current manufacturers have made modifications in their instruments allowing more efficient removal of bone with increased power. These devices are all more effective in performing the extensive sinus procedures currently being done with powered instrumentation.

TECHNOLOGY

Powered instrumentation in functional endoscopic sinus surgery has developed through an adaptation of surgical devices in broad use currently by orthopedic surgeons. These devices have been generically described as *soft tissue shavers,* as their main utility in orthopedic surgery is in the removal of tissue during arthroscopic procedure such as meniscectomy. While the term *shaver* is still used by many otolaryngologists to identify the powered devices, a term that is becoming more common currently is *microdebrider,* reflecting the use of a smaller version of the powered device in sinus surgery. In addition, the abandonment of the designation "soft tissue" reflects the current move to the performance of more bony dissection with these instruments. While Gross and Becker[7] take issue with the term *microdebrider,* we feel that this designation accurately describes both the design and function of the device, and will use this term throughout the present text.

All of these microdebrider devices have certain features in common. They all involve the use of a cutting bit consisting of a rotating inner cannula within a fixed outer housing (Figure 1.2). The bit has its cutting port on the lateral surface of the blade, with a small window toward the distal end of the device into which tissue is drawn. As the inner cannula rotates rapidly within the outer shaft, the tissue that has been drawn into the lumen is sheared off. The cutting bit is attached to a handpiece in which the motor that actuates the device is contained, and through which suction is supplied to the tip (Figure 1.3). The extracted tissue is then suctioned out of the device and into the table-side suction canister.

Critical to the operation of these microdebriders is sufficient suction pressure through the bit. The function of the device is dependent upon the tissue being drawn into the distal cutting port so that it can be sheared free. Various recommendations have estimated adequate suction pressures to be in the range of 180 mm Hg, although some of the more current models available require less suction pressure at the wall due to improved sealing mechanisms within the housing and handpiece. If the suction delivered is inadequate, the surgery will be technically frustrating and far less efficient.

Bit designs for the powered devices vary to some degree. All current bits involve blunt distal tips to prevent inadvertent penetration into structures distal to the tip. The cutting ports can incorporate differing edges for shearing the tissue, including razor-type and serrated edges. The outer diameter of the

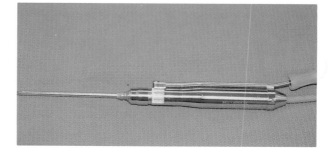

Fig. 1.3 Microdebrider handpiece with bit.

bits also varies, from 2.5 to 5.5 mm depending upon the manufacturer and the surgeon's preference. Smaller diameters are less efficient in the removal of bony material, and are far more prone to clogging with small bony fragments than are bits of greater diameter. In addition, bits can be straight, coaxial with the handpiece, or can have bends in the shaft of various contours and degrees. One manufacturer currently markets a malleable bit which can be manipulated by the surgeon at the time of the procedure to customize it for various applications. Bits can also vary in length from about 8 to 13.3 cm from their exit from the handpiece to their distal ends. While longer blades make surgery on the sphenoid sinus much more comfortable, there is a greater risk of perforation through the base of the skull and injury to critical structures with these longer bits.

An additional feature which is considered by some surgeons to be of use during sinus surgery is constant irrigation through the handpiece and microdebrider tip. It is the feeling of some otolaryngologists that this irrigation keeps the bit clean and results in less frequent clogging of the device by debris from the surgical field. In response to these suggestions, several manufacturers have decided to incorporate a constant irrigation mechanism into their microdebrider bits. Furthermore, an independent supplier has developed irrigating bits designed to retrofit handpieces made by the various manufacturers. While irrigation has some conceptual appeal to sinus surgeons, its true utility may well be exaggerated. In the hands of experienced surgeons, who occasionally rinse the device through by drawing in saline through the distal end intraoperatively, clogging is rarely a problem.

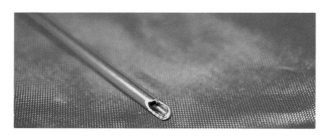

Fig. 1.2 Microdebrider cutting bits.

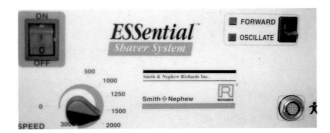

Fig. 1.4 Microdebrider power console.

The powered handpieces are controlled by a console placed off the surgical field, into which the handpieces are connected (Figure 1.4). These consoles allow adjustment of the speed of rotation of the bit, as well as changing the direction of the rotation from forward to backward, or allowing oscillation of the bit. Oscillation is felt to decrease clogging of the bit, and is the most frequently selected mode for operation. The motor is actuated through the use of a footpedal. These pedals also differ in design, and can involve simple pneumatic-controlled devices or electrical pedals which control not only actuation but direction and speed of rotation.

OUTCOME RESEARCH

The first discussion of the effectiveness of the powered technique for dissection of the paranasal sinuses was offered by Setliff and Parsons in 1994.[2] They described the effectiveness of the method in 345 patients. While the authors did not report their findings contrasting them to a group of patients who had undergone standard forceps-based functional endoscopic sinus surgery, it was their impression that the surgery was safe and effective in the removal of soft tissue disease and in various types of sinus procedures. They did report the exposure of orbital fat in one patient without significant consequence, and noted no significant postoperative complications in their sample. Setliff further comments on the safety of the procedure in a thorough discussion of his surgical approach to sinus disease.[8]

To date, the only scientific study to compare the effectiveness of the microdebrider technique for functional endoscopic sinus surgery with standard endoscopic procedures was reported by Krouse and

Christmas in 1996.[6] The study involved the examination of 250 patients who had undergone powered dissection of the sinuses, contrasting them with 225 patients who underwent nonpowered dissection using standard forceps-based principles. The study enrolled patients consecutively over a 2-year period, and included all patients on whom sinus surgery had been performed in the practices of the authors. The study was nonrandomized, but inclusive of all sinus patients during this period. Operative reports and office records were examined to assess a number of variables considered significant in evaluating the safety and efficacy of sinus surgical procedures. These variables included intraoperative bleeding, synechia formation postoperatively, lateralization of the middle turbinate, reocclusion of the maxillary ostium, symptom relief of patients postoperatively, and incidence of major complications. Table 1.1 displays the results.

In this study, it is clear that bleeding in the powered dissection group was markedly reduced compared to a forceps-based technique. In the use of forceps, removal of the tissue is accomplished through avulsion, even in the gentlest of hands. With powered instrumentation a sharp shearing effect is noted, cutting precisely across small vessels, and creating a seaming action which tends to decrease bleeding. In addition, postoperative complications were significantly reduced using the microdebrider for sinus surgery. No major complications such as orbital hematoma or cerebrospinal fluid leak were encountered in either group. Minor complications such as lateralization of the middle turbinate, postoperative synechia formation, and maxillary ostial

Table 1.1. Table title

	Microdebrider Group	Standard Group
Bleeding	19.5 cc	44.5 cc
Synechia formation	0 (0%)	4 (1.7%)
Lateralization	0 (0%)	5 (2.2%)
Ostial reocclusion	1 (0.4%)	7 (3.1%)
Average time to healing	39 days	55 days
Percent symptom-free	86%	87%
Major complications	0 (0%)	0 (0%)

From Krouse and Christmas.[6]

reocclusion were significantly reduced as well through the use of powered techniques. The authors also noted that the healing process was facilitated through this method, and that symptomatic relief in patients is equivalent between standard techniques and powered dissection. Krouse and Christmas conclude from this research that powered dissection of the paranasal sinuses is safe and effective, offers some advantages over traditional procedures on the paranasal sinuses in decreased bleeding, faster healing, and lesser postoperative complications.

Gross and Becker[7] report their experience with powered microdebriders in a 1996 article. The authors do not present any hard data, nor do they discuss the numbers of patients on whom they are basing their observations, but they do note that these devices have utility in a variety of circumstances. Gross and Becker find that powered techniques are especially useful in cases of severe polyposis, in sinusitis with subperiosteal abscess, and in revision sinus surgery. They report increased precision with the microdebrider, and decreased bleeding, particularly in cases in which excessive bleeding is anticipated.

Evidence from these various reports and studies supports the safety and efficacy of the powered technique in functional endoscopic sinus surgery. Sinus surgeons who have adopted this technique generally find surgery to involve significantly less bleeding, thereby increasing the safety and precision of the procedure. Normal tissue is able to be preserved, and decreased stripping of mucosa and lesser intraoperative trauma leads to faster healing with less postoperative complications. In addition, intraoperative time can be reduced up to 40% (personal communication, B. Manrin Rains, III, M.D., October 8, 1996). The weight of the evidence suggests that the use of powered instrumentation provides an important adjuvant modality to the concept of functional endoscopic sinus surgery as described by Kennedy[9] and Stammberger.[10] Additional research will continue to examine the precise role of this technique in sinus surgical procedures, and will likely see an expansion of this technology in otolaryngology.

REFERENCES

1. House WF, Hitselberger WE. Surgical complications of acoustic tumor surgery. *Arch Otolaryngol* 88:659–667, 1968.
2. Setliff RC, Parsons DS: The "Hummer": new instrumentation for functional endoscopic sinus surgery. *Am J Rhinol* 8:275–278, 1994.
3. Hawke WM, McCombe AW: How I do it: nasal polypectomy with an arthroscopic bone shaver: The Stryker "Hummer." *J Otolaryngol* 24:57–59, 1995.
4. Krouse JH, Christmas DA: Powered nasal polypectomy in the office setting. *Ear Nose Throat J* 75:608–610, 1996.
5. Christmas, DA, Krouse JH: Powered instrumentation in functional endoscopic sinus surgery I: surgical technique. *Ear Nose Throat J* 75:33–38, 1996.
6. Krouse JH, Christmas DA: Powered instrumentation in functional endoscopic sinus surgery II: a comparative study. *Ear Nose Throat J* 75:42–44, 1996.
7. Gross CW, Becker DG: Power instrumentation in endoscopic sinus surgery. *Oper Tech Otolaryngol Head Neck Surg* 7:236–241, 1996.
8. Setliff RC: The Hummer: a remedy for apprehension in functional endoscopic sinus surgery. *Otolaryngol Clin North Am* 29:98–104, 1996.
9. Kennedy DW, Zinreich SJ, Rosenbaum AE, et al: Functional endoscopic sinus surgery: theory and diagnostic evaluation. *Arch Otolaryngol* 111: 576–582, 1985.
10. Stammberger H: *Functional Endoscopic Sinus Surgery*. Philadelphia, Decker, 1991.

2

Endoscopic Anatomy of the Lateral Nasal Wall and Paranasal Sinuses

Eiji Yanagisawa, M.D., F.A.C.S.

The nasal cavity is divided by the median septum into two approximately symmetrical chambers. Each nasal cavity has an external or anterior opening (nare) and a posterior or pharyngeal opening (choana). The choana measures approximately 2.5 cm vertically and 1 cm transversely. Each nasal cavity consists of a medial wall (nasal septum), a lateral wall (nasal turbinates, meatus, and their contents), an inferior wall (floor), and a superior roof (cribriform plate).[1,2] A clear understanding of these structures is essential for the endoscopic sinus surgeon (Figures 2.1, 2.2).

Endoscopic examination of the nasal cavity should be carried out in a systematic fashion, as recommended by Stammburger and Kennedy.[3–5] The first pass is made along the floor of the nose between the nasal septum and the inferior turbinate using a 0 degree telescope. The anatomic structures to be observed are the inferior turbinate, the inferior meatus, the floor of the nose, the nasal septum, the eustachian orifice, and the nasopharynx. The second pass is made with the patient's head tilted backward approximately 45 degrees. The telescope is passed toward the middle turbinate and then advanced between the middle turbinate and inferior turbinate, visualizing the middle meatus and its contents such as the uncinate process, the ethmoidal bulla, the maxillary sinus ostia, and the hiatus semilunaris. If this anterior to posterior approach is impossible, the middle meatus and its contents may be examined by a posterior to anterior approach using a 30 degree or 70 degree telescope, first entering the wider posterior end of the middle meatus from below. The third

pass is directed toward the roof of the nasal cavity superiorly between the nasal septum and middle turbinate. The use of the 30 degree telescope may facilitate the examination of the roof of the nasal cavity and the sphenoid ostium in the sphenoethmoidal recess[1–29] (Figure 2.2).

In this chapter, pertinent endoscopic anatomy of the lateral wall of the nasal cavity and paranasal sinuses will be described. Anatomic terminology used in this chapter is based on the terminology of Stammberger et al (1995).[30]

ENDOSCOPIC ANATOMY OF THE LATERAL NASAL WALL

The lateral nasal wall consists of the nasal turbinates (inferior, middle, superior, and occasionally supreme), the meatus (inferior, middle, and superior), and their contents. The following are anatomic structures to be carefully observed.

Inferior Turbinate and Inferior Meatus

The inferior turbinate (Figures 2.1A, 2.2) is the largest of the three nasal turbinates. It has its own independent bone arising from the lateral wall of the nasal cavity articulating with the maxillary, lacrimal, palatal, and ethmoid bones. Its medial surface is usually concave and its lateral surface is convex. The turbinate is covered with a thick vascular membrane.[1,2] The hypertrophied inferior turbinate may occupy most of the anterior nasal cavity, making

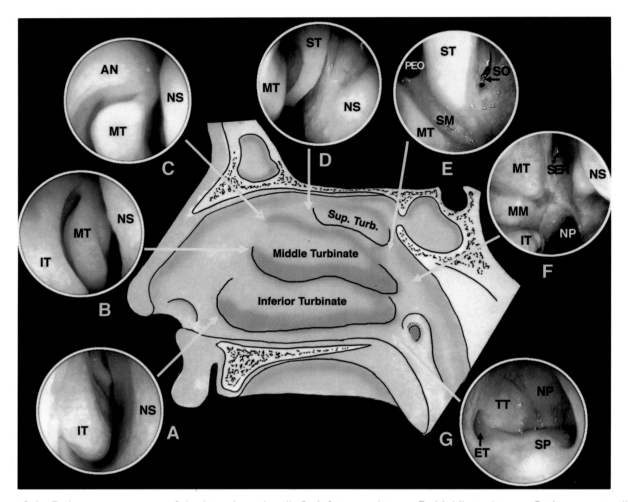

Figure 2.1. Endoscopic anatomy of the lateral nasal wall. **A:** Inferior turbinate. **B:** Middle turbinate. **C:** Agger nasi cell. **D:** Superior turbinate. **E:** Superior turbinate and superior meatus (PEO, posterior ethmoid sinus ostium, SO, sphenoid sinus ostium). **F:** Sphenoethmoidal recess (SER) and related structures (MT, middle turbinate; NS, nasal septum; MM, posterior nasal cavity and nasopharynx; ET, eustachian tube orifice; TT, torus tubarius; SP, soft palate). (From Yanagisawa E: *Color Atlas of Diagnostic Endoscopy in Otorhinolaryngology,* New York, Igaku-Shoin, 1996, p 43)

visualization of intranasal structures and the passage of a telescope often impossible. The application of nasal decongestants markedly decreases the size of the inferior turbinate, permitting passage of a telescope and visualization of intranasal anatomy and pathology.

The only significant anatomic structure of the inferior meatus is the ostium of the nasolacrimal duct (Figure 2.3). The lacrimal drainage system begins at the upper and lower puncta, which drain into the vertical, then the horizontal segments of the canaliculi in the common canaliculi and then enter the lacrimal sac. The lacrimal sac extends downward into the nasolacrimal duct, which travels in a bony canal along the medial maxillary wall until it opens into the inferior meatus through the valve of Hasner, located at the highest portion of the inferior meatus at the junction of the anterior and middle

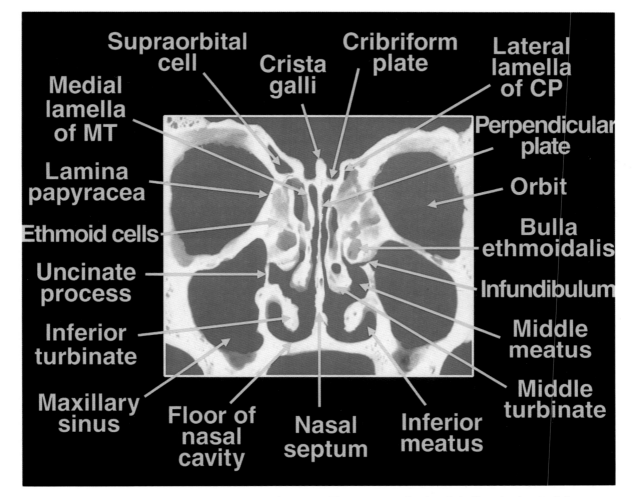

Figure 2.2. Anatomy of the nasal cavity and paranasal sinuses. This section of a dried skull at the level of the anterior ethmoid shows pertinent anatomic structures of the nasal cavities and paranasal sinuses. (From Yanagisawa E: *Color Atlas of Diagnostic Endoscopy in Otorhinolaryngology,* New York, Igaku-Shoin, 1996, p 42).

thirds of the meatus. The ostium lies 2.5 cm posterior to the anterior nasal sill.[7] The shape of the opening varies considerably from rounded to slit-like. When the opening is high, it tends to be wide; when it is located low, it is more apt to be slit-like.[2] Gentle digital pressure on the inner canthus usually expresses a few tears from the opening of the nasolacrimal duct. Recognition of this duct opening is important to prevent damage to the nasolacrimal

duct while performing an intranasal inferior meatal antrostomy.[5,30]

Middle Turbinate and Middle Meatus

Middle Turbinate

The middle turbinate (Figures 2.4 to 2.6), somewhat smaller than the inferior turbinate, is a part of the ethmoid bone covered by mucous membrane with

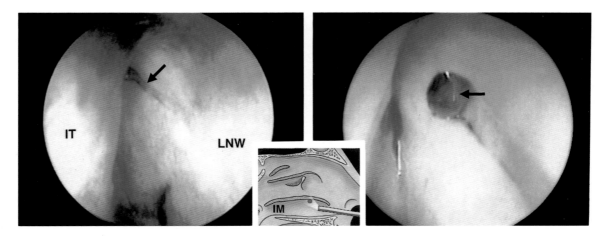

Figure 2.3. Inferior meatus and nasolacrimal duct. **A:** A 4-mm, 30 degree telescopic view of the inferior meatus showing the nasolacrimal duct (*arrow*). (IT, lateral aspect of the inferior turbinate; LNW, lateral nasal wall.) **B.** A close-up view with a 30 degree telescope clearly shows the opening of the nasolacrimal duct and a tear drop (*arrow*). (From Yanagisawa E: *Color Atlas of Diagnostic Endoscopy in Otorhinolaryngology,* New York, Igaku-Shoin, 1996, p 46).

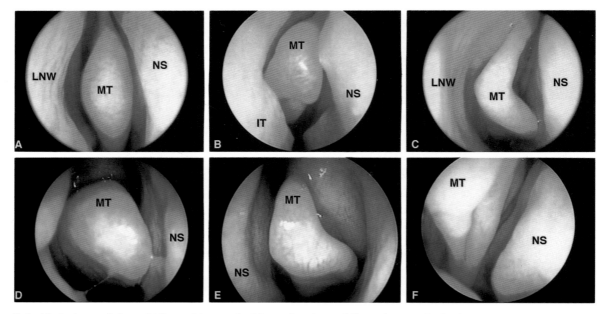

Figure 2.4. Variations of the middle turbinate. **A:** Normal right middle turbinate. **B:** Right middle turbinate with anterior polypoid mucosa. **C:** Medially (paradoxically) bent right middle turbinate. **D:** Concha bullosa. **E:** Triangular or L-shaped left middle turbinate. **F:** Sagittally clefted middle turbinate. Note the longitudinal cleft along the inferior border of the right middle turbinate. (From Yanagisawa E: *Color Atlas of Diagnostic Endoscopy in Otorhinolaryngology,* New York, Igaku-Shoin, 1996, p 47).

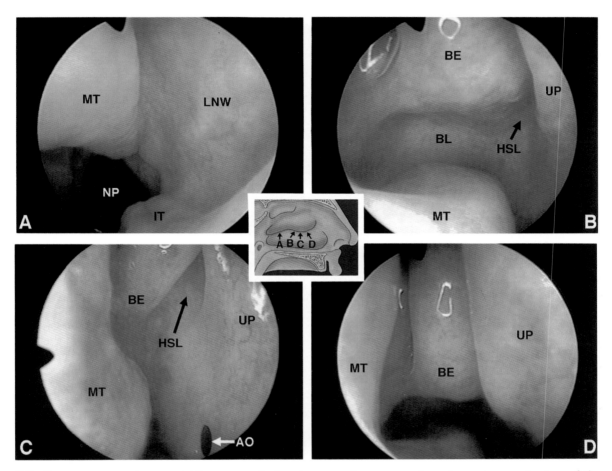

Figure 2.5. Structures seen in the middle meatus during the posterior to anterior telescopic examination of the middle meatus. **A:** Posterior third of the left middle meatus showing the posterior and ends of the middle (MT) and inferior (IT) turbinates, lateral nasal wall, and nasopharynx (NP). **B:** Middle third of the left middle meatus showing the ethmoid bulla (BE), laterally bent, horizontal lamella of the L-shaped left turbinate (MT), basal lamella (BL), middle turbinate (MT), hiatus semilunaris inferior (HSL), and uncinate process (UP). **C:** Midportion of the middle meatus showing the hiatus semilunaris inferior (HSL) between the inferior lateral portion of the ethmoid bulla (BE) and the uncinate process (UP). The lateral aspect of the middle turbinate (MT) is seen medially (MT), and the accessory maxillary sinus ostium is seen in the anterior interior portion of the lateral nasal wall (anterior fontanelle). **D:** Midportion of the middle meatus showing the anterior face of the ethmoid bulla (BE) between the middle turbinate (MT) and the uncinate process (UP). (From Yanagisawa E: *Color Atlas of Diagnostic Endoscopy in Otorhinolaryngology,* New York, Igaku-Shoin, 1996, p 49).

ciliated columnar epithelium. The anterior end of the middle turbinate has its own line of attachment running almost vertically upward to join the remainder of the turbinate at an angle or genu. The frontal recess is found beneath this genu. The frontal recess may receive the opening directly from the frontal sinus and the openings of some of the anterior ethmoid cells. The anterior third of the middle turbinate inserts vertically at the base of the skull at the lateral edge of the cribriform plate. The middle third of the middle turbinate is fixed to the lamina papyracea by its basal lamella, which runs in an

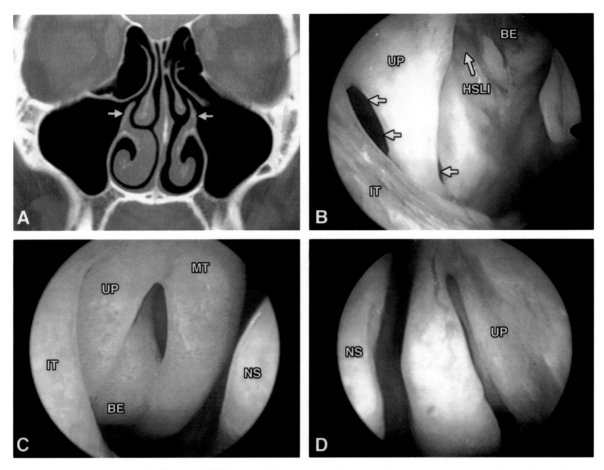

Figure 2.6. Uncinate process. **A:** Coronal CT scan of the sinuses showing the uncinate process (*arrow*) just below the ethmoid infundibulum forming a lateral wall of the middle meatus. **B:** Thirty degree telescopy of the lateral wall of the middle meatus showing the uncinate process (UP), hiatus semilunaris inferior (HSLI), ethmoid bulls (BE), and inferior turbinate (IT). The accessory maxillary sinus ostia are seen anterior to the uncinate process (anterior fontanelle) (*double arrows*) and posterior to the inferior portion of the uncinate process (posterior fontanelle) (*single arrow*). **C:** Zero degree telescopy showing a sickle-shaped uncinate process, prominent ethmoid bulla (BE) seen between the uncinate process (UP) and the middle turbinate (MT), inferior turbinate (IT) and the nasal septum (NS). **D:** Zero degree telescopy showing a medially bent left uncinate process narrowing the middle meatus. (From Yanagisawa E, Yanagisawa K: The uncinate process—a part of the ethmoid bone or the maxilla? *ENT J* 75:706–707, 1996.)

almost frontal plane. The posterior third of the middle turbinate is attached to the lamina papyracea and to the lateral wall of the nasal cavity. There are anatomic variations of the middle turbinate which include a triangular or L-shaped middle turbinate, a paradoxically bent middle turbinate, a concha bullosa, and a sagittal cleft of the inferior border of the

middle turbinate (Figure 2.4). Hyperpneumatization of the middle turbinate is known as the *concha bullosa*. It usually occurs bilaterally, but the degree of pneumatization may be variable. The presence of a concha bullosa is not necessarily a pathologic finding. However, if combined with an enlarged ethmoid bulla or a medially bent uncinate process, the concha bullosa can produce significant obstruction of the middle meatus, the hiatus semilunaris, and the ethmoid infundibulum. The middle turbinate converges toward the superior turbinate posteriorly, and its posterior end may be an important landmark when locating the sphenoid ostium in the sphenoethmoid recess. The main sphenoid sinus cavity is usually located superomedial to the posterior attachment of the middle turbinate. It is important to recognize the superior attachment of the middle turbinate to avoid injury to the cribriform plate.

Middle Meatus and Its Contents

The middle meatus (Figures 2.5 to 2.9), situated between the middle and inferior turbinates, contains many important anatomic structures essential for the endoscopic sinus surgeon. Anatomic structures to be recognized include the ethmoid bulla, the uncinate process, the hiatus semilunaris superior and inferior, the suprabullar or retrobullar recess (sinus lateralis), the frontal recess, the ethmoid infundibulum, the nasal fontanelles, the natural and accessory maxillary sinus ostia, and the ostiomeatal complex.

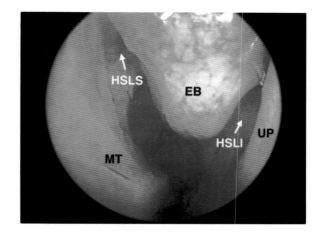

Figure 2.7. Hiatus semilunaris superior and inferior. Zero degree telescopy showing the hiatus semilunaris superior (HSLS) between the ethmoid bulls (EB) and the lateral wall of the middle turbinate (MT) and the hiatus semilunaris inferior in a groove between the ethmoid bulla (EB) and the uncinate process (UP). The hiatus semilunaris superior leads toward the frontal recess, while the hiatus semilunaris inferior leads toward the ethmoid infundibulum.

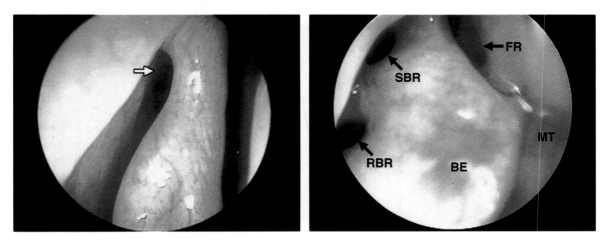

Figure 2.8. Frontal recess, suprabullar recess, and retrobullar recess. **A:** Zero degree telescopy demonstrates the right frontal recess (*arrow*) at the most superior portion of the middle meatus. **B:** Suprabullar and retrobullar recesses. Thirty degree telescopy of the superior portion of the right middle meatus shows the frontal recess (FR) openings of the suprabullar recess (SBR) and retrobullar recess (RBR), and the ethmoid bulla (BE).

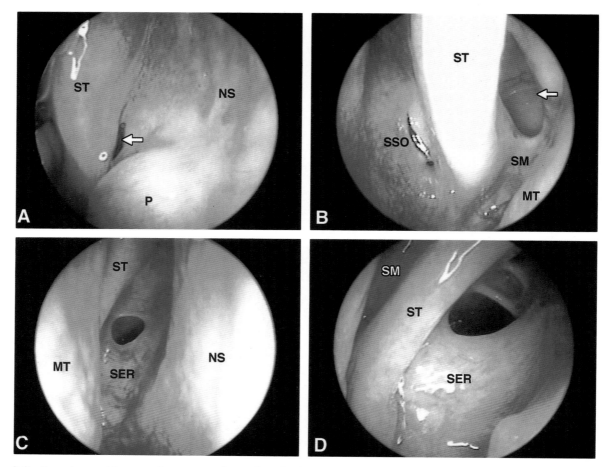

Figure 2.9. Superior turbinate and meatus, sphenoid, and ethmoid sinus ostia. **A:** Sphenoid sinus ostium. Zero degree telescopy shows the sphenoid sinus ostium in the sphenoethmoid recess between the posterior portion of the superior turbinate (ST) and the nasal septum (NS). Just below the ostium, a polyp (P) is seen. **B:** Superior meatus sphenoid sinus and posterior ethmoid sinus ostia. Zero degree telescopy shows a slit-like sphenoid sinus ostium (SSO) just medial to the posterior attachment of the superior turbinate (ST). A large ostium of the posterior ethmoid sinus is seen in the superior meatus (SM). A posterior ethmoid vessel can also be seen in the roof of the posterior ethmoid sinus (*arrow*). **C:** Sphenoid sinus ostium. Zero degree telescopy displays a sphenoid sinus ostium in the sphenoethmoid recess (SER) just medial to the posterior attachment of the superior turbinate (ST). Also seen are the middle turbinate on the left and the nasal septum on the right. **D:** Sphenoid sinus ostium. Close-up zero degree telescopy of the posterior superior right nasal cavity shows a large sphenoid sinus ostium in the sphenoethmoid recess (SER) just posterior and medial to the posterior attachment of the superior turbinate (ST). The superior meatus (SM) is also seen. (From Yanagisawa E: *Color Atlas of Diagnostic Endoscopy in Otorhinolaryngology,* New York, Igaku-Shoin, 1996, p 74)

Ethmoid Bulla (Bulla Ethmoidalis)

The ethmoid bulla (Figures 2.5 to 2.8) is a rounded prominence of the lateral wall of the middle meatus under cover of the middle turbinate. It consists of the largest and most nonvariant air cells in the anterior ethmoid complex. The bulla lamella forms the posterior wall of the frontal recess if it reaches the roof of the ethmoid. If it fails to reach the skull base, it results in formation of the suprabullar recess. The anterior wall of the ethmoid bulla is usually thin. This is an important landmark where anterior ethmoidectomy should begin either by a forceps or by a microdebrider.

Basal Lamella of the Middle Turbinate[30]

This structure is actually the third basal lamella of the ethmoturbinals (Figure 2.5). The insertion of the middle turbinate lies in three different planes. The anterior segment lies sagittally, attaching to the lateral end of the lamina cribrosa opposite its lamina lateralis. The middle segment is fixed to the lamina papyracea in an almost frontal plane. The posterior segment, called the *basal lamella,* is attached to the lamina papyracea, the medial wall of the maxillary sinus, or both to form the roof of the posterior third of the middle meatus.

The basal lamella of the middle turbinate divides the anterior and posterior ethmoid cells. It is an important landmark when performing posterior ethmoidectomy and sphenoidotomy.

Uncinate Process

The uncinate process (Figure 2.2 to 2.6) is a sickle-shaped, bony leaflet extending from its anterior superior attachment on the lateral nasal wall down to its posterior inferior attachment on the inferior turbinate. It extends posteromedially to its free margin. Its concave posterosuperior free margin is parallel to the anterior surface of the ethmoid bulla. The uncinate process attaches to the perpendicular process of the palatine bone and the ethmoid process of the inferior turbinate with bony spicules.[2–6,10–13,30] The convex anterior margin ascends to the lacrimal bone and sometimes to the skull base or the lamina papyracea, remaining in contact with the bony lateral nasal wall. The uncinate process may attach to the middle turbinate superiorly when curved medially in its superior most portion. When curved medially to a greater than usual extent, the free margin of the uncinate process may protrude into and sometime even out of the middle nasal meatus.[5,17,21,22,30]

Accessory Maxillary Sinus Ostium

The accessory maxillary sinus ostium (Figures 2.6, 2.10) is often visible in the lateral wall of the middle meatus by 0 and 30 degree telescopy. The accessory ostium may be encountered in 25–30% of the population. It is usually located in the anterior or posterior pontanelle, where the medial wall of the maxillary sinus is membranous. The size and shape of accessory ostia vary. The accessory ostium allows for recirculation whereby maxillary sinus secretions are passed out of the maxillary sinus via ciliary transport through the natural ostium and immediately back into the sinus via an accessory ostium.[2,5,8,10–12]

Nasal Frontanelle

The nasal fontanelle (Figure 2.6) is the area of the lateral wall of the middle meatus which is membranous without having a bony layer. The anterior fontanelle is anterior and inferior to the uncinate process, while the posterior fontanelle is posterior and superior to the uncinate process. The fontanelles are frequent sites of accessory maxillary sinus ostia.

Hiatus Semilunaris Superior and Inferior

The hiatus semilunaris inferior (Grünwald) is an anatomic plane that represents the shortest distance between the free posterior margin of the uncinate process and the corresponding anterior face of the ethmoid bulla (Figure 2.7). This is a passageway to the ethmoid infundibulum, which is a three-dimensional space. The hiatus semilunaris superior is a crescent-shaped cleft seen between the lateral surface of the middle turbinate and the superior portion of the ethmoid bulla leading toward the frontal recess. The hiatus semilunaris inferior is so named because it leads to the infundibulum and the maxillary sinus natural ostium, which are inferiorly positioned, while the hiatus semilunaris superior is so named because it leads to the frontal recess and the frontal sinus, which are superiorly situated.[20,29,30]

Frontal Recess

The frontal recess (Figure 2.8) is a most anterior and superior portion of the anterior ethmoid complex

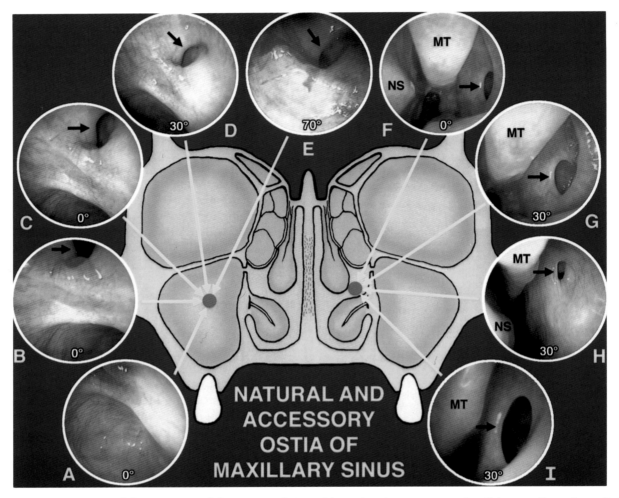

Figure 2.10. Overview of the anatomy of the paranasal sinus. Natural and accessory ostia of the maxillary sinus. **A:** Zero sinoscopic view of the right maxillary sinus via the canine fossa showing the posterior superior medial wall of the normal antrum. **B:** Zero degree sinoscopic view showing the right natural ostium coming into view. **C:** Further upward advancement of the zero degree telescope clearly reveals the natural ostium (*arrow*). **D:** Thirty degree sinoscopic view of the same natural ostium (*arrow*). **E:** Seventy degree sinoscopic view of the same maxillary sinus ostium. **F:** Accessory maxillary sinus ostium. Transnasal telescopic view of the accessory ostium of the left maxillary sinus. Zero degree telescopy shows an oval-shaped accessory ostium in the anterior fontanelle between the middle turbinate (MT) and the inferior turbinate. The nasal septum is seen medially. **G:** Accessory ostium. Thirty degree telescopy of the closer view of the same accessory ostium, as shown in part (F). **H:** Accessory ostium. Another 30 degree telescopy demonstrates the accessory ostium of the left maxillary sinus (*arrow*). **I:** The accessory ostium. Thirty degree telescopy gives the full view of a large accessory ostium. (From Yanagisawa E: *Color Atlas of Diagnostic Endoscopy in Otorhinolaryngology,* New York, Igaku-Shoin, 1996, p 68).

that leads to and communicates with the frontal sinus. It is seen as a recess in the most superior portion of the middle meatus. It is not the nasofrontal duct. The medial wall of the frontal recess is the most anterior and superior portion of the middle meatus. The lateral wall consists mostly of lamina papyracea. A discrete posterior margin exists only when the basal lamella of the bulla reaches the skull base separating the frontal recess from the suprabullar recess. This is an important landmark for endoscopic frontal sinus surgery.[5,30]

Suprabullar Recess and Retrobullar Recess

The suprabullar recess (Figure 2.8) is a space above the dome of the ethmoid bulla. It is often referred as the *sinus lateralis of Grünwald.* It should more appropriately called the *suprabullar recess* since this space does not have just one opening for ventilation and drainage and does not satisfy the criteria of a cell. The term *recess* is recommended by Stammberger et al.[30] The suprabullar recess may extend into a retrobullar recess when the posterior wall of the bulla lamella does not contact the basal lamella of the middle turbinate.

When pneumatized, this space is bordered superiorly by the ethmoid roof, laterally by the lamina papyracea, inferiorly by the roof of the ethmoid bulla, and posteriorly by the basal lamella of the middle turbinate. It is separated anteriorly from the frontal recess only when the bulla lamella reaches the skull base.[5,21,29,30]

Ethmoid Infundibulum

The ethmoid infundibulum (Figure 2.2) is a cleft or true three-dimensional space connecting the hiatus semilunaris inferior and the medial superior portion of the maxillary sinus. The ethmoid infundibulum is bordered medially by the uncinate process and laterally by the lamina papyracea.[30] At the superior end, the ethmoid infundibulum ends blindly in an acute angle, giving rise to the V-like-shape noted on the computed tomography (CT) scan. Posteriorly, the ethmoid infundibulum extends to the anterior face of the ethmoid bulla and opens into the middle meatus through the hiatus semilunaris inferior.

The frontal infundibulum is a funnel-shaped narrowing of the inferior aspect of the frontal sinus toward the floor of the frontal sinus ostium. It is located inside the frontal sinus.

The maxillary infundibulum is the funnel-shaped narrowing of the lumen of the maxillary sinus toward its natural ostium. Typically, the lumen does not narrow significantly toward the maxillary sinus ostium.

Ostiomeatal Complex (OMC)

The ostiomeatal complex, often mistakenly spelled as *osteomeatal,* is a functional entity of the anterior ethmoid complex that represents the final common pathway for drainage and ventilation of the frontal, maxillary, and anterior ethmoid cells. When any or all cells, clefts, and ostia in the middle meatus are involved in a disease process, it will lead to sinusitus. This space is bounded by the middle turbinate medially, the lamina papyracea laterally, and the basal lamella superiorly and posteriorly. The inferior and anterior borders of OMC are open. This space contains the agger nasi cells, nasofrontal recess, infundibulum, bulla ethmoidalis, and anterior ethmoid cells.[3,4,10]

Superior Turbinate and Superior Meatus

The superior nasal turbinate (Figures 2.1D, E and 2.9; see also Figure 2.15) is short, only about half of the length of the middle turbinate. The superior meatus is a narrow channel between the superior turbinate and the posterior half of the middle turbinate. Most posterior ethmoid air cells open into this meatus (Figure 2.9).

The supreme nasal turbinate, when present, is usually a rather slight fold. The shallow groove below it is the supreme meatus and is said to receive the ostium of posterior ethmoid cells. The part of the nasal cavity between the uppermost turbinate superior or supreme and the anterior surface of the body of the sphenoid bone is the sphenoethmoidal recess. The ostium of the sphenoid sinus is typically through the posterior wall of this recess (Figure 2.9).

ENDOSCOPIC ANATOMY OF THE PARANASAL SINUSES

Endoscopic anatomy of the maxillary, ethmoid, frontal, and sphenoid sinuses and their ostia will be briefly described.

Maxillary Sinus (Antrum of Highmore)

The maxillary sinus (Figures 2.2, 2.10–2.12) is usually the largest of the paranasal sinuses situated in the body of the maxilla. Its medial wall is the lateral wall of the nasal cavity, its anterior wall is the facial surface of the maxilla, its posterior wall is the anterior wall of the pterygomaxillary fossa, and its floor is the alveolar and palatine processes of the maxilla. The average dimensions of the maxillary sinus in adults are a height of 33 mm, a width of 23 mm, and a depth of 34 mm.[1,2]

Accessory Maxillary Sinus Ostium

An accessory maxillary sinus ostium (Figures 2.6, 2.10) can be seen in the lateral wall of the middle meatus in approximately 25–30% of the population. It is usually located in the anterior or posterior fontanelle, where the medial wall of the maxillary sinus is membranous. The size and shape of the

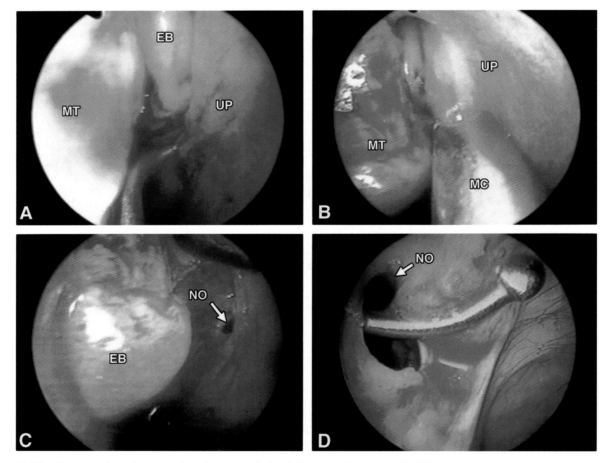

Figure 2.11. Transnasal endoscopic localization of the left natural ostium. **A:** The posterior free edge of the uncinate process just anteromedial to the ethmoid bulla (EB) is identified and retracted anteriorly. **B:** The posterior free edge of the uncinate process is excised with a back-biting forceps and/or a microdebrider, exposing the hiatus semilunaris inferior and the ethmoid infundibulum where the left natural maxillary sinus ostium (NO) is located. The ethmoid bulla is seen medial to this groove. **C:** The Lusk maxillary sinus probe is passed through this natural ostium into the maxillary sinus. **D:** Maxillary sinoscopy via the canine fossa clearly demonstrates the probe passed through the natural ostium seen transnasally.

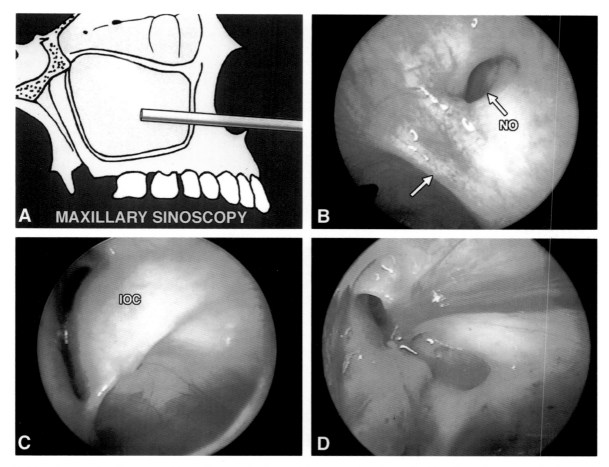

Figure 2.12. Transcanine fossa maxillary sinoscopic view of the natural ostium. **A:** Maxillary sinoscopy via the canine fossa. **B:** Thirty degree sinoscopy showing the right natural ostium in the medial, superoposterior portion of the maxillary sinus (NO). The prominent mucosal ridge is constantly seen just inferior to the natural ostium. **C:** Infraorbital ethmoid cell (Haller's cell). Zero degree maxillary sinoscopy shows the infraorbital ethmoid cell narrowing the maxillary infundibulum and the natural ostium. **D:** Thirty degree maxillary sinoscopy reveals the blood-tinged mucus being transported into the lower portion of the natural ostium of the left maxillary sinus.

accessory ostia vary, as seen in Figure 2.10. It may be roundish or oval. There may be two or more accessory ostia. The accessory ostium allows for recirculation whereby maxillary sinus secretions are passed out of the maxillary sinus via ciliary transport through the natural ostium and immediately back into the sinus via an accessory ostium. For this reason, the accessory ostium encountered during endoscopic sinus surgery should be connected to the natural ostium to prevent mucus recirculation.[5,8,19]

Natural Maxillary Sinus Ostium

The natural maxillary sinus ostium (Figures 2.10–2.12) is located within the ethmoid infundibulum, which is hidden by an intact uncinate process and usually cannot be visualized transnasally. Only when the posterior free margin of the uncinate process is removed does the natural ostium become visible (Figure 2.11).

The most common site of the natural ostium is in the posterior third of the ethmoid infundibulum

(31.8%). The ostium is found in the anterior third in 5.5% of the population and in the middle third in 11%. In 11.6% of specimens, the ostium was at the extreme posterior tip of the infundibulum.[31]

When the natural ostium is viewed transantrally via the canine fossa by maxillary sinoscopy, the natural ostium is usually found in the posterosuperior portion of the medial wall of the maxillary sinus (Figure 2.12). The ostium is usually single, and its shape may be slit-like, spindle, or triangular. Often it looks like a canal. Almost always there is an oblique or horizontal thick mucosal fold beneath the ostium (Figures 2.11D, 2.12B). The ostium is best seen with a 30 degree telescope. When the 0 degree telescope is used, it is necessary to tilt and direct the tip of the telescope posterosuperiorly. Other structures to be recognized by maxillary sinoscopy include an infraorbital ethmoid cell (Haller's cell, an extension of the inferior ethmoid cell into the medial portion of the roof of the maxillary sinus); an accessory ostium found in the medial sinus wall; an infraorbital canal containing a neurovascular bundle seen in the roof of the sinus; and bony elevations by teeth roots in the floor of the sinus. Streaking of the blood-tinged mucus (mucociliary flow) into the natural ostium may be seen during maxillary sinoscopy[5,8,29]) (Figure 2.9D).

Ethmoid Sinus

The ethmoid sinus (Figures 2.2, 2.13) consists of a variable number of ethmoid air cells that honeycomb the ethmoid bone and lie between the upper part of the lateral nasal wall and the medial wall of the orbit (lamina papyracea). The basal lamella of the middle turbinate divides the anterior ethmoid air cells from those of the posterior ethmoid. Ethmoid air cells may invade the frontal bone, the maxilla, or the sphenoid bone. The average dimensions of the ethmoid sinuses are approximately 5 cm in depth, approximately 3 cm in height, and approximately 0.5 cm in width anteriorly and 1.5 cm posteriorly. Usually, the posterior ethmoid cells open into the superior meatus[2] (Figure 2.9B), while the anterior ethmoid cells drain into the ethmoid infundibulum. The agger nasi is the most superior remnant of the first ethmoturbinal, which persists as a mound or crest immediately anterior and superior to the insertion of the middle turbinate. An agger nasi cell results when this area of the lateral nasal wall undergoes pneumatization.[1,2,30]

During endoscopic ethmoidectomy, the following structures should be carefully identified to prevent serious complications: the superolateral wall of the middle turbinate; the lateral lamella of the cribriform plate; the lamina papyracea; the roof of the ethmoid sinuses; and the anterior and posterior ethmoid arteries.

Lateral Lamella of the Cribriform Plate

The lateral wall of the superior vertical portion of the middle turbinate attaches to the skull base and may constitute the medial wall of the completed endoscopic ethmoidectomy. The lateral lamella of the cribriform plate lies just above the superior attachment of the middle turbinate (Figure 2.13C, D). This lateral lamella may protrude into the ethmoid cavity and form the superior medial portion of the ethmoid sinus (Figure 2.13C, D). This area becomes vulnerable to surgical trauma when the disease within the frontal recess and the ethmoid sinus is removed. This structure should be carefully studied by preoperative coronal CT scans.[14,16,29,30]

Anterior and Posterior Ethmoid Arteries

The anterior ethmoid artery (Figure 2.13C) is an important anatomic landmark for the roof of the ethmoid sinuses or the anterior skull base. The anterior ethmoid artery, a branch of the ophthalmic artery, leaves the orbit via the anterior ethmoidal foramen, crosses the roof of the anterior ethmoid sinus, and supplies the anterior ethmoid and frontal sinuses. The artery then enters the anterior cranial fossa and thereafter turns downward into the nasal cavity through the slit by the side of the crista galli. The anterior ethmoidal artery is distributed to the anterior third of the lateral wall of the nasal cavity and to a similar portion of the nasal septum. The anterior ethmoid artery is normally much larger than the posterior ethmoid artery.[2,5,9,15]

Both anterior and posterior ethmoid foramina are usually situated along the frontoethmoid suture line, as seen in the medial wall of the orbit (Figure 2.13A). The distance between the anterior and posterior ethmoidal foramina averages 10 mm.[1,9] The distance from the posterior ethmoidal foramen to the

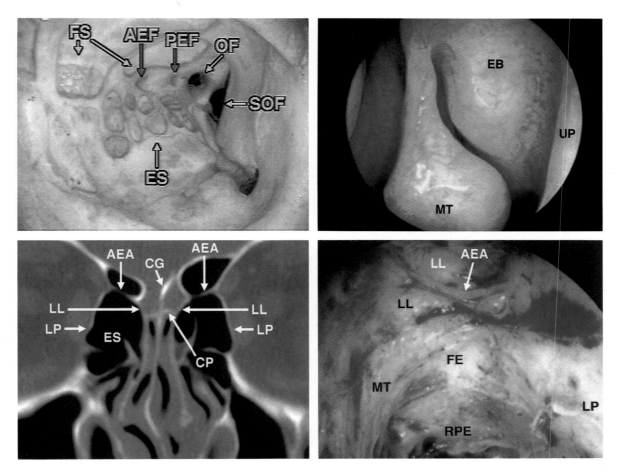

Figure 2.13. Ethmoid bulla, lateral lamella of the cribriform plate, and anterior ethmoid artery. **A:** Medial wall of the left orbit. Dried skull demonstrates the frontal sinus (FS), anterior ethmoid foramen (AEF), posterior ethmoid foramen (PEF), optic foramen (OF), superior orbital fissure (SOF), lamina papyracea, and exposed ethmoid sinus (ES). **B:** Ethmoid bulla. Zero degree telescopy reveals a prominent ethmoid bulla (EB) between the middle turbinate (MT) and the uncinate process (UP). **C:** Lateral lamella of the cribriform plate. Coronal CT scan of the sinuses shows clearly the lateral lamella of the cribriform plate (LL) protruding into the superomedial portion of the ethmoid sinuses (ES). Anterior ethmoid canal containing the anterior ethmoid artery (AEA) and nerve is well shown crossing the superior portion of the ethmoid sinus between the lateral lamella of the cribriform plate and the superomedial wall of the orbit. The can also shows a paper-thin lamina papyracea (LP), ethmoid sinus (ES), and crista galli (CG). **D:** Ethmoid sinus. Zero degree telescopic view of the superior portion of the left ethmoid sinus after complete ethmoidectomy showing the lateral lamella of the cribriform plate (LL), anterior ethmoid artery (AEA), fovea ethmoidalis (FE), attachment of the vertical portion of the middle turbinate to the base of the skull (MT), roof of the posterior ethmoid sinus (RPE), and the lamina papyracea (LP). The frontal racess is situated just anterior and superior to the anterior ethmoid artery. (From Ohnishi T, Yanagisawa E: Lateral lamella of the cribriform plate—an important high-risk area in endoscopic sinus surgery. *ENT J* 74:688–690, 1995.)

anterior portion of the optic foramen is 4–7 mm in 84% of the skulls studied by Kirchner et al.[9] Figure 2.13D shows the roof of the ethmoid cavity following completion of endoscopic ethmoidectomy on the left side. The anterior ethmoid artery is seen traveling in a thin-walled, bony canal beneath the roof of the ethmoid sinus and between the lateral and medial walls of the ethmoid sinus. Unless the artery is recognized, it can be easily injured during surgery. As shown in Figure 2.13D, there are bony protrusions at the medial and lateral ends of the anterior ethmoid bony canal containing the artery and the nerve. Injury to these protrusions may lead to cerebrospinal fluid leakage, orbital hematoma, or intracranial infections.[14,15] The weakest point of the entire anterior base of the skull is that point at which the anterior ethmoid artery leaves the ethmoid and enters the ethmoidal sulcus of the olfactory fossa, usually referred as the *lateral lamella of the cribriform plate*. Seventy percent of the bony canal of the anterior ethmoid artery lies just below the skull base and 30% lies above the roof of the skull base.[9]

According to Stammberger, one way to find the anterior ethmoid artery by the endoscopic approach is to follow the anterior ethmoid bulla in the direction of the roof of the ethmoid. If the bulla lamella extends up to the roof of the ethmoid, the ethmoidal artery can usually be found immediately adjacent to this point, usually 1 to 2 mm posteriorly.[5]

The anterior ethmoid artery serves as an important landmark for the entrance to the frontal recess, which begins just anterior to this artery.

Lamina Papyracea

The lamina papyracea, a paper-thin medial of the orbit, forms the lateral wall of the ethmoid sinus (Figure 2.13A,C,D). Trauma to this thin wall may result in protrusion of the orbit fat. This is one of the most common sites of injury during ethmoidectomy. Palpation of the eyeball on the side of the injury may result in further protrusion of the bloody fatty tissues into the ethmoid cavity, confirming the tear of the lamina papyracea (Stankiewicz's maneuver).

Ethmoid Bulla

The ethmoid bulla is a hollow, thin-walled, bony prominence and consists of the largest and most nonvariant air cells in the anterior ethmoid complex (Figures 2.5B–D, 2.13B). It is formed by pneumatiza-

tion of the bulla lamella. Its size and shape may be quite variable. This is an important landmark where the anterior ethmoidectomy should begin.

Infraorbital Ethmoid Cell (Haller's Cell)

This is an anterior ethmoid air cell which has grown into the bony orbital floor that constitutes the roof of the maxillar sinus (Figure 2.12C). This may narrow the ethmoid infundibulum and/or the natural maxillary sinus ostium.

Onodi Cell (Sphenoethmoid Cell)

The Onodi cell is the most posterior and superior cell of the posterior ethmoid sinus, which extends into the superolateral portion of the sphenoid sinus. The optic nerve and carotid artery may be exposed in the Onodi cell. This is clinically significant because the sphenoid sinus is located medially and inferiorly to the most posterior cell of the posterior ethmoid complex. Consequently, an attempt to use instrumentation to locate the sphenoid sinus directly behind the last cell of the posterior ethmoid complex may result in serious trauma to the optic nerve or carotid artery in the presence of the Onodi cell.[5,30]

Frontal Sinus

Usually there are two paired frontal sinuses in the anterior portion of the frontal bone. They are separated by a bony septum located approximately in the midline. However, asymmetry of the frontal sinuses is common. The ostium of the frontal sinus is in the posteromedial part of the sinus floor, usually at the lowest point of the floor (Figure 2.14). The ostium may open directly into the frontal recess. The lumen of the ostium is often narrowed by expansion of the surrounding anterior ethmoid cells or by the enlargement of the middle turbinate. Van Alyea describes two major types of frontal drainage. He found that in 86% of the patients the frontal sinus drained anterior to, superior to, or posterior to the ethmoid infundibulum.[32] In the other 14%, the frontal sinus drained directly into the infundibulum.

The inside of the frontal sinus may be visualized by intranasal frontal sinoscopy via the frontal recess or by external frontal sinoscopy via the anterior wall

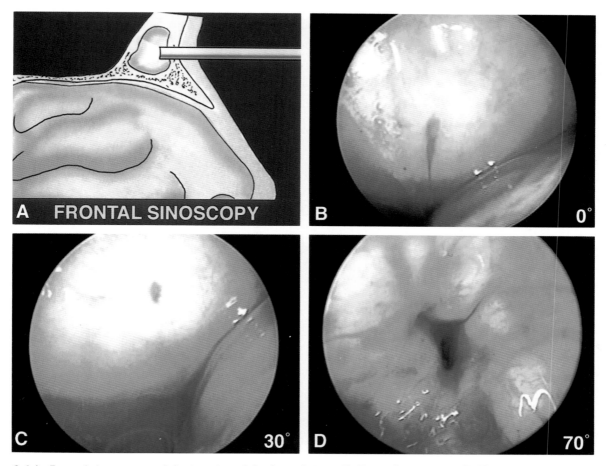

Figure 2.14. Frontal sinoscopy and the interior of the frontal sinus. **A:** Frontal sinoscopy . **B:** Zero degree frontal sinoscopy shows the edematous mucosa of the posterior wall of the sinus and the glimpse of the frontal sinus ostium. **C:** Thirty degree frontal sinoscopy shows inferior portion of the frontal sinus. **D:** Seventy degree frontal sinoscopy shows the frontal sinus ostium in the posteromedial portion of the floor of the frontal sinus.

or floor of the frontal sinus. Frontal sinoscopy using 0, 30, and 70 degree telescopes allows the study of anatomy and pathology of the frontal sinus (Figure 2.14).

Sphenoid Sinus

The sphenoid sinuses (Figures 2.9, 2.15) are usually contained within the body of the sphenoid bone and, in many cases, are divided into two sinuses by a septum in the midline. The two sphenoid sinuses are rarely symmetrical in size and shape. There may be more than one septum dividing the sinuses into

several compartments. The sphenoid sinus is often invaded by posterior ethmoidal cells. Pneumatization of the sphenoid sinus may extend superolaterally into the lesser ring of the sphenoid and the anterior clinoid process; laterally into the greater wing of the sphenoid; inferolaterally into the pterigoid process (Figure 2.15D); and anteroinferiorly into the posterior portion of the nasal septum. Several structures can bulge into the sphenoid sinus: the optic nerve and the internal carotid artery in the superolateral wall (Figure 2.15B, C), the maxillary nerve in the lateral wall, and the canal of the vidian nerve in the floor of the sinus.

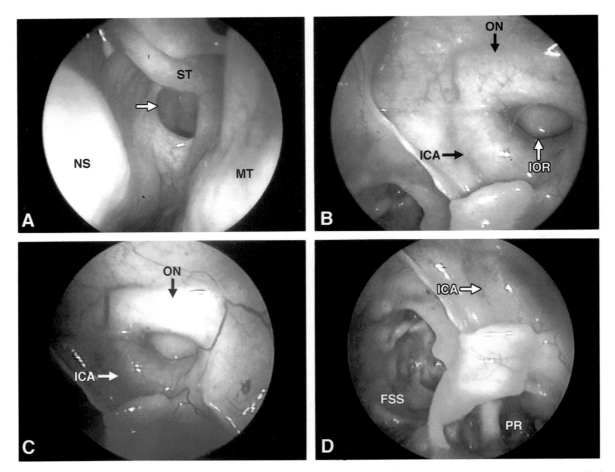

Figure 2.15. Sphenoid sinus and its contents. **A:** Sphenoidotomy opening. Zero degree telescopy reveals a widely patent left sphenoidotomy opening (*arrow*) in the sphenoethmoidal recess inferolateral to the left superior turbinate (ST). **B:** Optic nerve and internal carotid artery. Zero degree telescopy of the sphenoid sinus through the sphenoidotomy opening shows the optic nerve (ON) and exposed internal carotid artery (ICA) in the superolateral wall of the sphenoid sinus. The recess between the structures is an infraoptic recess (IOR). **C:** Optic nerve and internal carotid artery. Thirty degree telescopy directed laterally within the left sphenoid sinus clearly shows the optic nerve (ON) and the internal carotid artery (ICA). **D:** The internal carotid artery and the pterygoid recess. Thirty degree telescope directed inferiorly within the left sphenoid sinus demonstrates the main cavity of the sinus and its floor (FSS) medially, the internal carotid artery (ICA) superolaterally, and the pterygoid recess (PR) inferolaterally. (From Yanagisawa E: *Color Atlas of Diagnostic Endoscopy in Otorhinolaryngology,* New York, Igaku-Shoin, 1996, p 75)

Sphenoid Sinus Ostium

The sphenoethmoidal recess lies in the angle between the ethmoid bone and the anterior surface of the sphenoid bone. The sphenoid sinus ostium (Figure 2.9) is usually located in the posterior wall of this recess. The distance from the nasal spine to the anterior wall of the sphenoid sinus is approximately 7 cm. Endoscopically, the sphenoid sinus ostium can be found in the sphenoethmoidal recess medial to the superior or supreme turbinate in the superoposterior portion of the nasal cavity and lateral to the posterosuperior portion of the nasal septum (Figure 2.9). The shape of the ostium may vary widely, appearing slit-like, round, or oval. It should be remembered that the sphenoid sinus ostium opens in the superior portion of the anterior wall of the sphenoid sinus approximately 15 mm from the floor of the sinus. When enlarging the ostium, the surgeon should remember that the main sphenoid sinus cavity is inferior to this ostium.

Optic Nerve and Internal Carotid Artery

The endoscopic sinus surgeon should always remember the anatomic location of the optic nerve and the internal carotid artery within the sphenoid sinus (Figure 2.15B, C). They lie in the superior and lateral wall of the sphenoid sinus. In the presence of an Onodi cell, the most posterosuperior cell of the posterior ethmoid sinuses which invades the sphenoid sinus and surrounds the optic nerve (present in 10% of cases), the optic nerve may be enclosed within the Onodi cell.

When sphenoidotomy is performed via the posterior ethmoid sinus, the sphenoid sinus should be entered as medially and inferiorly as possible to avoid injuries to the optic nerve and internal carotid artery. When the anterior wall of the sphenoid sinus cannot be identified, it is best to find the natural ostium of the sphenoid sinus in the sphenoethmoidal recess medial to the superior turbinate and enlarge the sphenoid sinus ostium inferiorly and medially. The bony canal covering the internal carotid artery may be partially dehiscent (25% of cases).[5,26,30] Inadvertent injury to these structures may result in blindness and catastrophic hemorrhage.

REFERENCES

1. Gray H: *Anatomy of the Human Body.* Philadelphia, Lea & Febiger, 1966.
2. Hollinshead WH: *Anatomy for Surgeons. The Head and Neck.* New York, Harper & Row, 1968.
3. Kennedy DW: Functional endoscopic sinus surgery—technique. *Arch Otolaryngol* 111:643–649, 1985.
4. Kennedy DW, Zinreich SJ, Rosenbaum AE, et al: Functional endoscopic sinus surgery. *Arch Otolaryngol* 111:576–582, 1985.
5. Stammberger H: *Functional Endoscopic Sinus Surgery: The Messerklinger Technique.* Philadelphia, BC Decker, 1991.
6. Anand VK, Panje WR: *Practical Endoscopic Sinus Surgery.* New York, McGraw-Hill, 1993.
7. Calhoun KH, Rotzer WH, Stiernberg CM: Surgical anatomy of the lateral nasal wall. *Otolaryngol Head Neck Surg* 1032:156–160, 1990.
8. Draf W: Therapeutic endoscopy of the paranasal sinuses. *Endoscopy* 10:247–254, 1078.
9. Kirchner JA, Yanagisawa E, Crelin ES: Surgical anatomy of the ethmoidal arteries: a laboratory study of 150 orbits. *Arch Otolaryngol* 74:382–386, 1961.
10. Levine HL, May M: *Endoscopic Sinus Surgery.* New York, Thieme, 1993.
11. Mehta D: *Atlas of Endoscopic Sinonasal Surgery.* Philadelphia, Lea & Febiger, 1993.
12. Messerklinger W: *Endoscopy of the Nose.* Baltimore, Urban & Schwartzenberg, 1978, pp 1–178.
13. Rice DH, Schaeffer SD: *Endoscopic Paranasal Sinus Surgery,* 2nd ed. New York, Raven Press, 1993.
14. Ohnishi T, Tachibana T, Kaneko Y, et al: High-risk areas in endoscopic sinus surgery and the prevention of complications. *Laryngoscope* 103:1181–1185, 1993.
15. Ohnishi T, Yanagisawa E: Endoscopic anatomy of the anterior ethmoid artery. *ENT J* 73:634–636, 1994.
16. Ohnishi T, Yanagisawa E: Lateral lamella of the cribriform plate—an important high-risk area in endoscopic sinus surgery. *Ear Nose Throat J* 74:688–690, 1995.
17. Wigand ME: *Endoscopic Surgery of the Paranasal Sinuses and Anterior Skull Base.* New York, Thieme Verlag Stuttgart, 1990.
18. Yanagisawa E, Yanagisawa K: Endoscopic view of ostium of nasolacrimal duct. *Ear Nose Throat J* 72:491–492, 1993.
19. Yanagisawa E, Yanagisawa K: Endoscopic view of maxillary sinus ostia. *Ear Nose Throat J* 72:518–519, 1993.
20. Yanagisawa E, Weaver EM: Endoscopic view of the hiatus semilunaris superior and inferior. *Ear Nose Throat J* 75:460–462, 1996.
21. Yanagisawa E, Weaver EM: Endoscopic view of

the suprabullar and retrobullar recesses (sinus lateralis). *Ear Nose Throat J* 75:578–579, 1996.

22. Yanagisawa E: Endoscopic view of the medially bent uncinate process. *Ear Nose Throat J* 75:648, 656, 1996.

23. Yanagisawa E, Yanagisawa K: The uncinate process—a part of the ethmoid bone or the maxilla? *Ear Nose Throat J* 75:706–707, 1996.

24. Yanagisawa E: Endoscopic view of the middle turbinate. *Ear Nose Throat J* 72:725–727, 1993.

25. Yanagisawa E, Weaver EM: Anatomical variations of the middle turbinate. *Ear Nose Throat J* 75:194–197, 1996.

26. Yanagisawa E: Endoscopic view of sphenoethmoidal recess and superior meatus. *Ear Nose Throat J* 72:331–332, 1993.

27. Yanagisawa E: Endoscopic view of sphenoid sinus cavity. *Ear Nose Throat J* 72:393–394, 1993.

28. Yanagisawa E, Yanagisawa K: Endoscopic view of exposed vital structures following sphenoethmoidectomy. *Ear Nose Throat J* 73:810–811, 1994.

29. Yanagisawa E, Yanagisawa R: *Color Atlas of Diagnostic Endoscopy in Otorhinolaryngology.* New York, Igaku-Shoin, 1996.

30. Stammberger HR, Kennedy DW, et al. Paranasal sinuses: anatomic terminology and nomenclature. *Ann Otol Rhinol Laryngol* 104(Suppl 167: 7–16, 1995.

31. Van Alyea OE: Maxillary sinus drainage. *Ann Otol Rhinol Laryngol* 55:754–763, 1946.

32. Van Alyea OE: Frontal sinus drainage. *Ann Otol Rhinol Laryngol* 55:267–277, 1946.

3

Radiologic Anatomy of the Paranasal Sinuses

Ramón E. Figueroa, M.D.

Whether classic functional endoscopic sinus surgery (FESS) or powered endoscopic sinus surgery (PESS), surgical treatment planning requires a thorough understanding of paranasal sinus anatomy as shown by modern computed tomography (CT). Meticulous attention to scanning protocols and patient preparation is required to achieve the degree of accurate detailed information needed for safe and effective surgery.

CT PROTOCOLS

The complete evaluation of paranasal sinus anatomy requires imaging planes perpendicular to the structures of surgical interest. Due to the complex anatomy of this region, both coronal and axial scanning planes are necessary. The ostiomeatal complex, agger nasi region, and cribriform plate are best demonstrated in the coronal plane. The axial plane is best suited for evaluation of the frontal recess and frontal sinus, the sphenoethmoidal recess, and the anatomic relationship between the sphenoid sinuses, the internal carotid arteries, and the optic nerves.

PATIENT PREPARATION

The imaging goal should always be to depict the underlying anatomic problem that is causing recurrent sinus disease. To achieve this goal, it is imperative that patients are treated with antibiotics and decongestants in order to eliminate all reversible disease prior to their imaging studies. Clear anatomic landmarks and/or disease that persists in spite of treatment will dictate the site and extent of surgical intervention needed.

COMPLETE SINUS CT

This CT technique is used specifically for presurgical evaluation in patients with recurrent episodes of sinusitis in spite of adequate medical treatment. The presurgical evaluation for PESS is achieved with the patient in supine position, using continuous axial 3-mm images along the plane of the hard palate, covering from the floor of the maxillary sinus to the top of the frontal sinus. The coronal study is performed with the patient in prone position (to displace any residual sinus fluid away from the maxillary sinus ostium) using continuous 3-mm images perpendicular to the hard palate, covering from the nasofrontal suture to the posterior wall of the sphenoid sinus (Figure 3.1). The images are obtained with bone algorithm and low photon techniques (80–100 milliamp) to decrease the radiation exposure to the cornea of the patient. Filming parameters should emphasize resolution of air–mucosa–bone boundaries, achieved in most scanners by printing the images with a wide window (@2,000 Hounsfield units) and a negative level (−200). The coronal images should be also printed in soft tissue windows

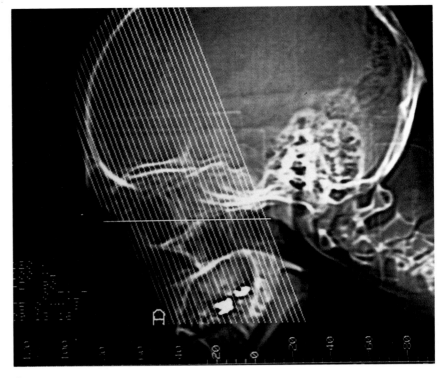

A

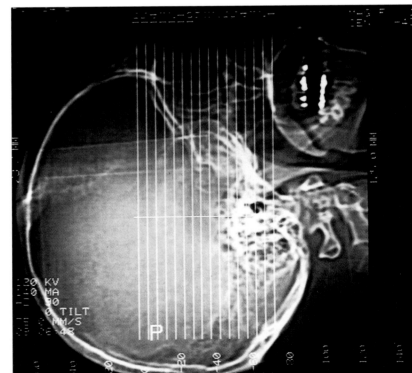

Figure 3.1. Complete sinus CT. **A:** Contiguous 3-mm coronal images are perpendicular to hard palate, from frontal to sphenoid sinus, with the patient in prone position. **B:** Axial images are oriented along the long axis of the hard palate to cover from the palate to the top of the frontal sinus, with patient in supine position. (Figueroa RE, Kuhn FA: Imaging evaluation for functional endoscopic sinus surgery. In Taveras J, Ferrucci R (eds.): *Radiology: Diagnosis, Imaging, Intervention.* Philadelphia, JB Lippincott, 1995, Chapter 12B. Reprinted with permission of the author.)

B

(W: 350, L: 50) to evaluate adjacent soft tissue structures. Modern CT scanning techniqes also allow generation of high-quality sagittal reformatted images from the axial or coronal data sets. Three-dimensional images and computer-based "image layers" could also be created in a computer workstation to rehearse a difficult surgery prior to the actual procedure. This technique is particularly useful when planning additional surgery in patients who have extensive scarring and loss of anatomic landmarks due to previous unsuccessful surgeries.

LIMITED SINUS CT

Initial evaluation of acute sinusitis and follow-up evaluations of patients with chronic sinusitis do not require the detailed complete sinus CT examination used for surgical planning; they could be performed with an abbreviated, quicker and less expensive technique. This "screening" or "limited sinus CT" consists of six axial 3-mm CT images obtained at equal distances, oriented parallel to the hard palate, followed by six coronal 3-mm CT images perpendicular to the hard palate (Figure 3.2). Low photon scanning and wide window printing techniques are performed as in the complete sinus CT. The limited sinus CT is intended to replace the complete sinus x-ray series previously used for sinusitis evaluation, providing better quality of information for patient management. A word of caution at this time is appropriate. The limited sinus CT does not provide a complete anatomic evaluation of the sinuses and should not be used for surgical planning of endoscopic procedures. It is to be used only for evaluating acute disease or response to treatment.

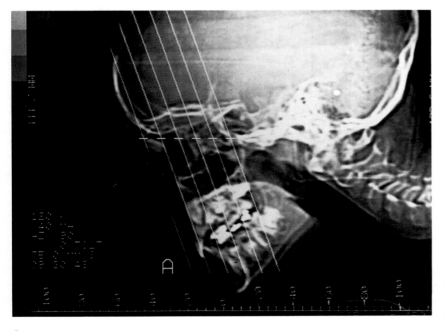

A

Figure 3.2. Limited sinus CT. **A:** Six equally spaced coronal images are prescribed from frontal to anterior sphenoid sinus, with patient in prone position.

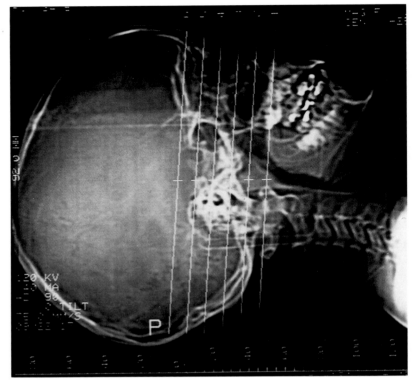

Figure 3.2. B: Six equally spaced axial images are prescribed from the floor of the maxillary sinus to the midfrontal sinus. For patients unable to be scanned in prone position, closer spaced axial images and coronal reformatted images could be used as an option. (Figueroa RE, Kuhn FA: Imaging evaluation for functional endoscopic sinus surgery. In Taveras J, Ferrucci R (eds): *Radiology: Diagnosis, Imaging, Intervention.* Philadelphia, JB Lippincott, 1995, Chapter 12B. Reprinted with permission of the author.)

B

FUNCTIONAL ANATOMY OF PARANASAL SINUSES

The paranasal sinuses are the respiratory system's first line of defense against external insult. In addition to warming and humidifying the air we inhale, the nasal mucosa traps in its mucous blanket most of the bacteria, viruses, allergens, and other noxious agents that are transported by inspired air. This mucous blanket is created by the goblet cells of the nasal mucosa and transported by its columnar ciliary epithelium. The mucociliary blanket thus created is carried by the cilia toward the natural ostium of each sinus, where it empties through the ostiomeatal complex or the sphenoethmoidal recess into the nasopharynx. Anatomic variants or pathol-ogy that narrows drainage pathways could produce repetitive episodes of sinus secretion accumulation behind the points of stenosis or obstruction. Sinusitis could occur when infectious agents from the nasal cavity secondarily grow in these accumulated secretions.

Ostiomeatal Complex

The anterior paranasal sinus complex is composed of the frontal sinuses, the agger nasi cells, anterior ethmoidal labyrinth, supraorbital ethmoidal cells (when present), and maxillary sinuses. Secretions from these sinus spaces empty into a sagittally oriented sickle-shaped space within the lateral nasal wall known as the ethmoidal infundibulum (Figure 3.3). The ethmoidal infundibulum starts anterior-

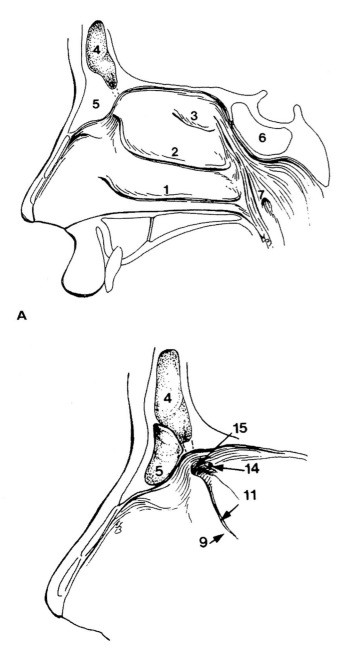

A

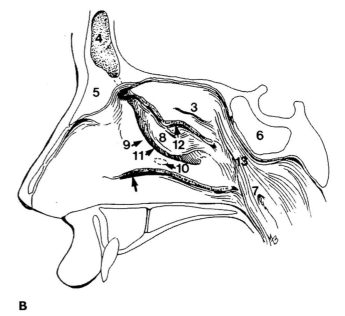

B

C

Figure 3.3. Anatomy of the lateral nasal wall. **A:** Line diagram view from the nasal septum. **B:** Lateral nasal wall after removal of inferior and middle turbinates exposes the components of the ostiomeatal complex. Long arrow points to the opening of the nasolacrimal duct in the inferior meatus (valve of Hasner). **C:** Detail of frontal recess, agger nasi cell, and position of anterior ethmoidal artery at the posterior margin of the frontal recess. 1. inferior turbinate; 2. middle turbinate; 3. superior turbinate; 4. frontal sinus, with natural ostium in intermittent line; 5. agger nasi cell; 6. sphenoid sinus; 7. torus tubarius; 8. bulla ethmoidalis; 9. uncinate process; 10. outlined maxillary sinus natural ostium behind uncinate process; 11. hiatus semilunaris; 12. sinus lateralis under the basal lamella of middle turbinate; 13. sphenoethmoidal recess; 14. anterior ethmoidal artery position; 15. frontal recess. (Figueroa RE, Kuhn FA: Imaging evaluation for functional endoscopic sinus surgery. In Taveras J, Ferrucci R (eds): *Radiology Diagnosis, Imaging, Intervention.* Philadelphia, JB Lippincott, 1995, Chapter 12B. Reprinted with permission of the author.)

superiorly at the frontal recess below the natural ostium of the frontal sinus, courses inferior-posteriorly medial to the lamina papyracea of the orbit, hidden from the nasal cavity by the mucosal reflection of the uncinate process. Secretions within the three-dimensional space of the ethmoidal infundibulum empty into the nasal cavity through the hiatus semilunaris inferioris, a two-dimensional "door" defined by the distance between the free edge of the uncinate process and the bulla ethmoidalis (Figure 3.4). The ethmoidal infundibulum terminates at the posterior margin of the hiatus semilunaris above the posterior

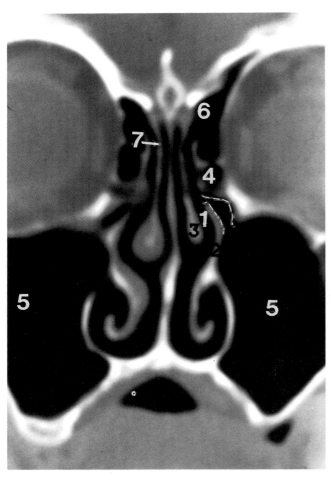

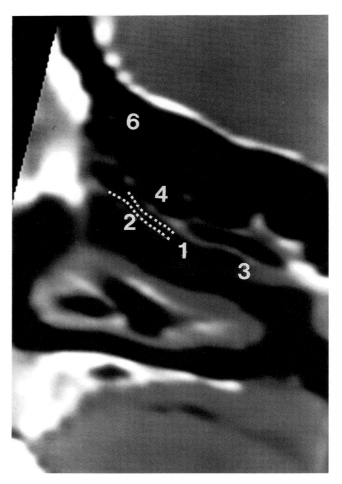

A   B

Figure 3.4. Ostiomeatal complex (OMC). **A:** Coronal CT in mucosal windows shows the ethmoidal infundibulum (*dotted lines*) behind the uncinate process (2), the middle meatus (1), middle turbinate (3), bulla ethmoidalis (4), maxillary sinuses (5), frontal recess (6) and vertical attachment of the middle turbinates (7). **B:** Sagittal reformatted image from coronal CT shows the hiatus semilunaris opening (*dotted lines*) between the free edge of the uncinate process (2) and the bulla ethmoidalis (4). (Figueroa RE, Kuhn FA: Imaging evaluation for functional endoscopic sinus surgery. In Taveras J, Ferrucci R (eds): *Radiology: Diagnosis, Imaging, Intervention.* Philadelphia, JB Lippincott, 1995, Chapter 12B. Reprinted with permission of author.)

third of the inferior turbinate. It is defined laterally by the lamina papyracea of the orbit, inferomedially by the uncinate process and posterosuperiorly by the bulla ethmoidalis. The bulla ethmoidalis is the largest, most constant anterior ethmoidal cell, arising from the lamina papyracea and projecting toward the middle meatus. Its attachment, the bulla lamella, could extend to the skull base or fuse laterally to the lamina papyracea, creating a narrow space between its upper margin and the basal lamella of the middle turbinate known as the sinus lateralis. The opening of the sinus lateralis toward the middle meatus is known as the hiatus semilunaris superioris.

Secretions from the frontal sinus, agger nasi cells, and anterior ethmoid sinus drain into the superior portion of the ethmoidal infundibulum. On the other hand, the maxillary sinus secretions are carried by mucociliary transport through its natural ostium in the superior portion of its medial wall, opening low into the junction of the middle and posterior thirds of the ethmoidal infundibulum. All these secretions empty into the middle meatus and are carried by mucociliary transport toward the nasopharynx anterior to the torus tubarius. The combination of the lamina papyracea, uncinate process, bulla ethmoidalis, and the middle turbinate, with the spaces defined by them (ethmoidal infundibulum, hiatus semilunaris inferioris, and middle meatus) integrate the functional concept known as the ostiomeatal complex. This region is best evaluated in the coronal CT images. Special attention is given to the caliber of the ostiomeatal complex spaces, which could be narrowed by nasal septal deformities and spurs, paradoxical middle turbinates, or pneumatization of the middle turbinates (concha bullosa), large bulla ethmoidalis, Haller cells, or ethmoidal pneumatization of the inferior lamina papyracea at the maxillary ostium (Figure 3.5).

An especially difficult anatomic area is the frontal recess, where the frontal sinus natural ostium assumes a funnel shape downwards, emptying through the frontal recess into the upper ethmoidal infundibulum. The lateral nasal wall nasofrontal junction area is known as the agger nasi mound, which projects anterior and slightly inferior to the frontal recess. Whenever there is agger nasi pneuma-

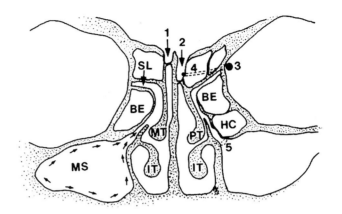

Figure 3.5. Paranasal coronal anatomy and variants. **A:** Line diagram shows normal ostiomeatal anatomy on the right side and variants on the left side. Notice the normal mucociliary pattern of drainage of the right maxillary sinus into the ethmoidal infundibulum, the natural ostium of the left maxillary sinus (5), the sinus lateralis (SL), the shallow right (1) and the deep left (2) olfactory fossae. The course of the left anterior ethmoidal artery (4) from the ophthalmic artery (3) to the lateral lamella of the cribriform plate could cross the anterior ethmoidal labyrinth or the frontal recess. Other structures shown are the bulla ethmoidalis (BE), Haller cell (HC), paradoxical middle turbinate (PT), inferior (IT) and middle (MT) turbinates. (Figueroa RE, Kuhn FA: Imaging evaluation for functional endoscopic sinus surgery. In Taveras J, Ferrucci R (eds): *Radiology: Diagnosis, Imaging, Intervention.* Philadelphia, JB Lippincott, 1995, Chapter 12B. Reprinted with permission of the author.)

tization, the frontal recess will be proportionately elevated, and even stenosed by hyperpneumatized agger nasi cells (Figure 3.3C). This area is carefully best evaluated combining the axial and the coronal CT images around the nasofrontal suture and in sagittally reformatted images obtained from the axial data set (Figure 3.6A, B).

Sphenoethmoidal Recess

The functional unit for the posterior paranasal sinus is the sphenoethmoidal recess. This is a gutter-like depression in the lateral nasal wall posterior to the

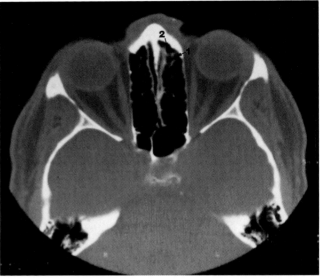

Figure 3.6. Frontal recess anatomy. **A:** Axial image at the agger nasi level shows the left frontal recess (1) bordered anteriorly by an agger nasi cell (2). **B:** Sagittal reformatted image from the axial data shows the elevation of the left frontal recess (1) by the agger nasi cell (2). Notice the frontal sinus (3), anterior ethmoidal labyrinth (4), and sphenoethmoidal recess (5).

A

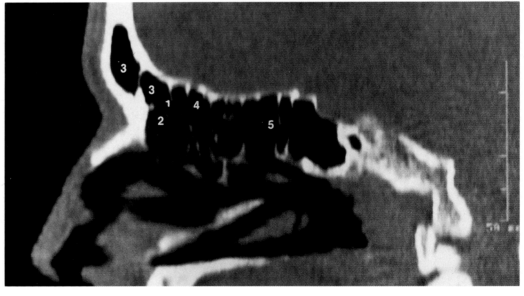

B

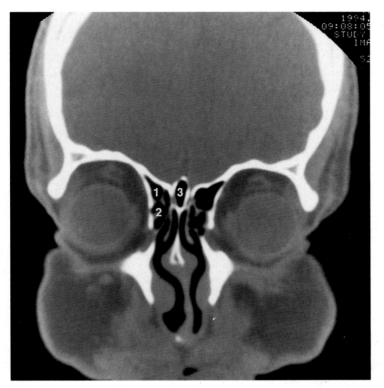

Figure 3.6. C: Coronal image of other patient shows the typical position of the agger nasi cell (2) anterior to the uncinate process in the lateral nasal wall. Notice the left frontal recess (1) and the pneumatized crista galli (3).

superior turbinate and anterior to the face of the sphenoid sinus. It channels the secretions arising from the sinuses located posterior to the basal lamella of the middle turbinate: the posterior ethmoid and sphenoid sinuses. These secretions are transported by mucociliary action posterior to the torus tubarius down toward the nasopharynx. The sphenoethmoidal recess is best demonstrated in axial projections, defined by the posterior extent of the nasal septum as it merges with the sphenoid sinus wall (Figure 3.7). The natural ostium of each sphenoid sinus is easily identified opening into the sphenoethmoidal recess, also acting as a reliable anatomic marker. The posterior ethmoid sinus drains through the superior meatus into the sphenoethmoidal recess approximately opposite the sphenoid sinus ostium. Mucosal lesions or enlarged adenoidal lymphoid tissue could selectively impair sphenoethmoidal recess drainage, in which case patients present with predominant posterior sinusitis.

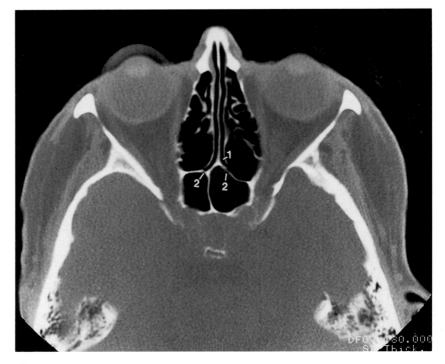

A

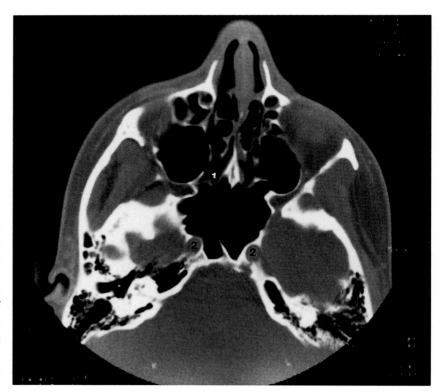

Figure 3.7. Sphenoethmoidal recess and sphenoid sinus. **A:** Axial image shows the divergent space of the sphenoethmoidal recess (1) along the sides of the posterior nasal septum as it meets the rostrum of the sphenoid sinus. Notice the natural ostia of the sphenoid sinuses (2). **B:** Sphenoid sinus can hyperpneumatize, outlining adjacent structures along its walls. Notice the sphenoethmoidal recess (1), the asymmetric intersinus septum, and the bulging internal carotid arteries posteriorly (2).

B

36

SURGICAL DANGER ZONES

Frontal Recess and Anterior Ethmoidal Artery

The anterior ethmoidal artery is a distal branch of the ophthalmic artery, which crosses the lamina papyracea within the posterior wall of the frontal recess to penetrate the lateral lamella of the cribriform plate, finally supplying the olfactory mucosa and the anterior end of the falx cerebri. Occasionally, the anterior ethmoidal artery projects within the frontal recess, covered by a thin bony canal or dehiscent of bone cover, outlined only by mucosa. This anatomic variant, recognizable on coronal 3-mm CT (Figures 3.5A, 3.8B), poses a risk of arterial hemorrhage or acute orbital bleed in surgical exploration of the frontal recess.

Ethmoidal Labyrinth and Olfactory Fossa

The roof of the ethmoidal labyrinth is formed by the frontal bone and its fovea ethmoidalis, which provide a thick protective barrier to internal ethmoidectomy instrumentation. However, the medial wall of the anterior ethmoidal labyrinth is formed by the lateral lamella of the cribriform plate, a thin wafer of bone that defines the lateral margin of the olfactory fossa. The length of the lateral lamella of the cribriform plate is dictated by how deep the olfactory fossa projects into the nasal cavity (Figures 3.5, 3.8A–C). Stammberger classified the olfactory fossa in three types. Type 1 is described as the shallow olfactory fossa where the cribriform plate is at or just below the level of the fovea ethmoidalis of the frontal bone. Type 2 refers to the olfactory fossa where the length of the lateral lamella and the cribriform plate are similar, with a squared symmetric olfactory fossa lateral to the crista galli; and Type 3 is identified as the deep olfactory fossa in which the length of the lateral lamella is greater than the length of the cribriform plate. Type 3 olfactory fossae project deep into the nasal cavity and are potential sources of inadvertent intracranial penetration and cerebrospinal fluid leaks whenever there is medial migration of surgical dissection and lateral lamella perforation during internal ethmoidectomy procedures.

Uncinate Process, Haller Cells, and Lamina Papyracea

Haller cells are created by ethmoidal pneumatization of lamina papyracea medial to the natural ostium of the maxillary sinus, and, if large, could potentially impair drainage of the maxillary sinus (Figure 3.9A, B). The presence and specific location of Haller cells is to be documented in the presurgical CT, since this cell is hidden from view by the uncinate process, and is frequently missed on nasal endoscopic examination. The surgical resection of Haller cells requires a three-dimensional awareness of its relationship with the lamina papyracea and the orbit to avoid orbital penetration during an endoscopic procedure. Dehiscence of the lamina papyracea and prolapses of orbital fat into sinus spaces are also important to recognize presurgically in the complete sinus CT examination (Figure 3.9C).

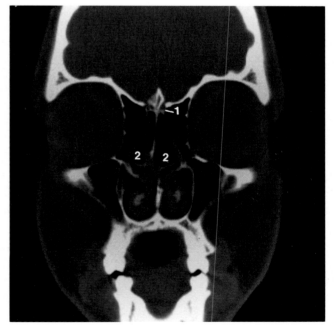

A

Figure 3.8. Olfactory fossa and anterior ethmoidal artery. **A:** Type I shallow olfactory fossa shows a short lateral lamella of the cribriform plate (1). Notice also the bilateral concha bullosae (2).

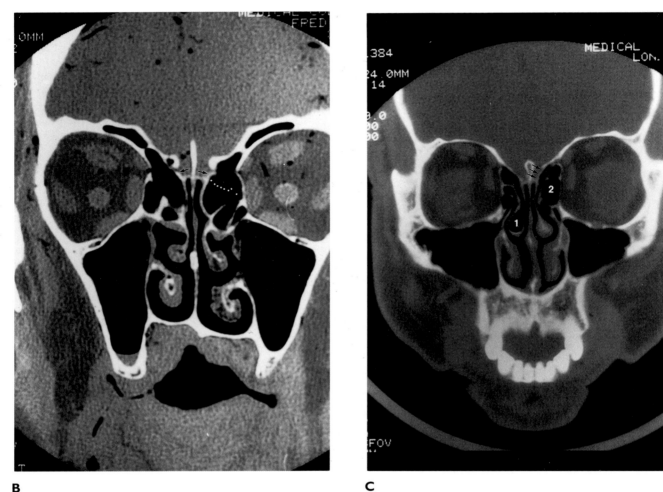

B   **C**

Figure 3.8. **B:** Cadaver coronal image at the frontal recess shows a dehiscent left anterior ethmoidal artery crossing from the orbit to the olfactory fossa (*dotted line*). Type 2 olfactory fossa shows its lateral lamella of similar length as the ipsilateral cribriform plate (*arrowheads*). **C:** Type 3 olfactory fossa shows its lateral lamella longer than the ipsilateral cribriform plate, projecting deeper into the nasal cavity (*small arrows*). Notice a right concha bullosa (1) and a large left bulla ethmoidalis (2).

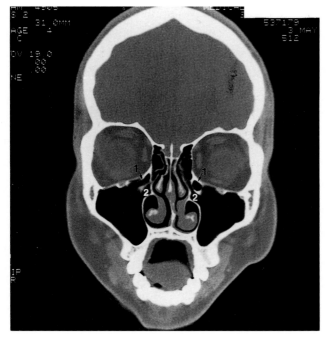

A

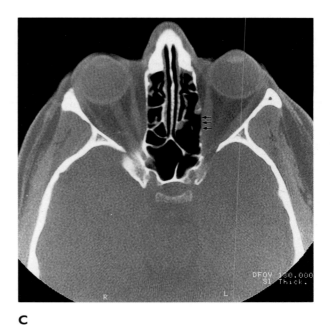

C

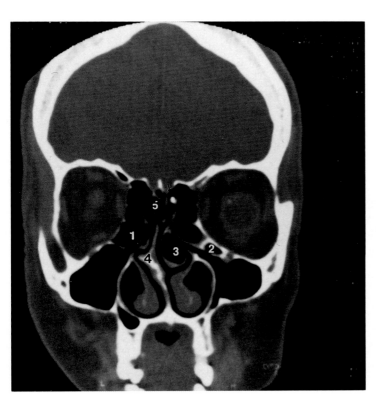

B

Figure 3.9. Haller cell and lamina papyracea. **A:** Bilateral Haller cells (1) along the inferior medial orbital wall could narrow the natural ostium of the maxillary sinuses (2). **B:** Large right bulla ethmoidalis (1) and left Haller cell (2) compromise the drainage pathways of the maxillary sinuses. The left concha bullosa (3) narrows the left middle meatus. The nasal septum is deviated to the right, with a nasal spur (4) impinging at the base of the right inferior turbinate. Notice a small ethmoidal osteoma (*arrow*) and pneumatized superior turbinates (5). **C:** Dehiscence of the lamina papyracea is a potential source for iatrogenic complication during PESS internal ethmoidectomies, recognized as an area of air–orbital fat interface (*arrows*).

This understanding is of special importance in PESS, where the vacuum-assisted powered blade could suction a sizable volume of orbital fat and contents before the surgeon is aware this has happened. Gentle technique and leaving the patient's ipsilateral eye uncovered during surgery should help prevent or minimize this complication.

Uncinate Process and Nasolacrimal Duct

CT is ideal for defining the thickness of (or absence of) bone covering the nasolacrimal duct, as well as its proximity to the uncinate process (Figure 3.10). A thick bone buttress between these two structures should protect the nasolacrimal duct during powered uncinectomies, since most powered bits lack enough torque to easily shave thick bone. An initial uncinate incision with a backbiter or similar instrument is required to provide an edge for the suction bit to start the uncinectomy. Recognition of a dehiscent nasolacrimal duct or thin bone covering this duct is important to prevent the uncinate incision or subsequent aggressive PESS uncinectomy from cre-

ating a nasolacrimal fistula or secondary nasolacrimal duct adhesions.

Onodi Cells and Optic Nerves

The posterior ethmoid sinus could pneumatize posteriorly above the sphenoid rostrum, extending laterally toward the clinoid processes. This pattern of pneumatization is known as Onodi cells. Whenever present, Onodi cells tend to expose the optic nerves submucosally along their superior lateral wall, creating a zone of potential iatrogenic injury when Onodi cell penetration occurs during transethmoidal sphenoidotomy (Figure 3.11).

Sphenoid Sinus, Optic Nerves, and Internal Carotid Arteries

As a general rule, the sphenoid sinuses are asymmetric, with the intersinus septum frequently projecting off midline depending on the pattern of sinus pneumatization. The sphenoid sinus frequently

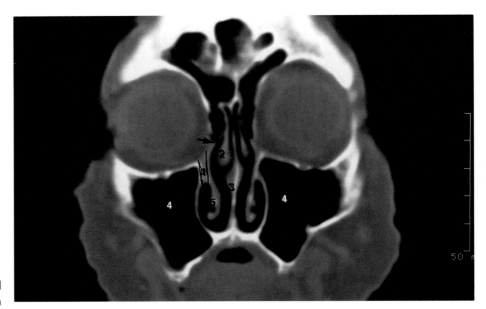

Figure 3.10. Nasolacrimal duct and uncinate process. **A:** Coronal 3-mm CT image.   **A**

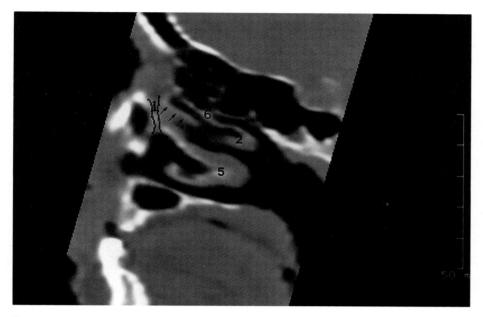

B

Figure 3.10. B: Sagittal reformatted image from coronal CT data. These images shows the vertical orientation of the nasolacrimal duct (1) from the lacrimal sac to the valve of Hasner at the inferior meatus. Notice the close anatomic relationship of the uncinate process (*arrows*) and the nasolacrimal duct (outlined 1). Other nearby structures are middle turbinate (2), nasal septum (3), maxillary sinus (4), inferior turbinate (5), and the basal lamella of the middle turbinate (6).

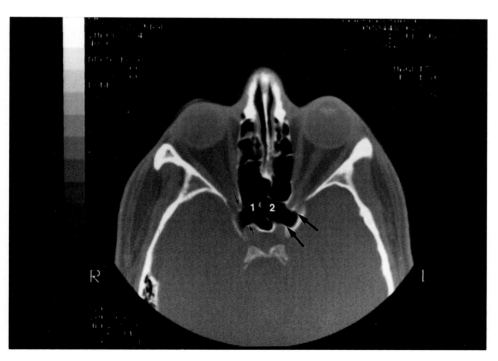

A

Figure 3.11. Onodi cells and optic nerves. **A:** Axial image shows right ethmoidal Onodi cell (1) pneumatizing posteriorly, outlining the right optic nerve (*small arrows*). The left sphenoid sinus pneumatizes the left clinoid process, with the left optic nerve outlined by mucosa (*large arrows*).

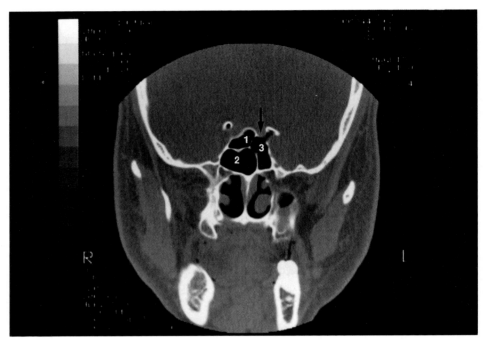

Figure 3.11. B: Coronal image shows the Onodi cell (1) above the right sphenoid sinus (2). Notice the dehiscent left optic nerve (*arrow*) above the left sphenoid sinus (3).

B

hyperpneumatizes, extending into the pterygoid plates, posterior nasal septum, into the dorsum sella or the clivus. This hyperpneumatization could produce areas of bone dehiscence, which could expose the optic nerves, the maxillary nerve (V2), or the internal carotid artery in submucosal position, leaving these structures vulnerable to inadvertent surgical trauma in sphenoid sinus instrumentation. Axial CT images tend to better depict the anatomic rela-tionship of the pneumatized sphenoid sinus with the optic nerves and internal carotid arteries, showing as two bulges in the lateral wall of the sphenoid sinus (Figure 3.12). Coronal CT images are also needed to define the sellar floor relationship to the sphenoid sinus septum, optic nerves, and internal carotid arteries in cases of transsphenoidal hypophysectomy in which the rhinologist creates the surgical approach for the neurosurgical procedure.

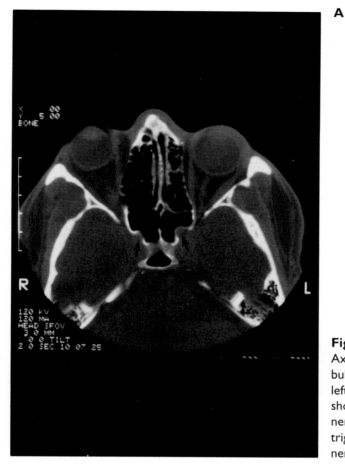

A

Figure 3.12. Sphenoid sinus and internal carotid arteries. **A:** Axial image shows the internal carotid arteries producing focal bulges (*arrows*) on the sphenoid sinus posterior walls, with the left internal carotid artery partially dehiscent. **B:** Coronal image shows the anatomic relationships of the sphenoid sinus: optic nerves (1), internal carotid arteries (2), maxillary division of the trigeminal nerve within the foramen rotundum (3), and vidian nerve (4).

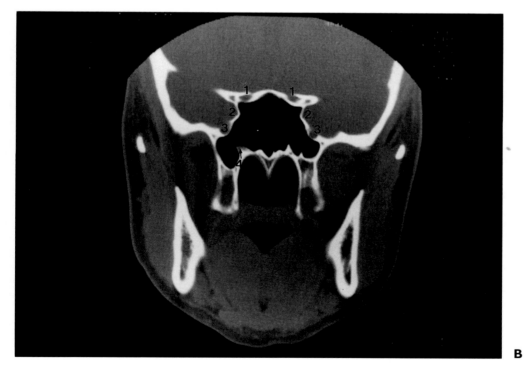

B

SELECTED READINGS

Babbel R, Harnsberger HR, Nelson B, et al: Optimization of techniques in screening CT of the sinuses. *AJR* 157:1093–1098, 1991.

Bolger WE, Butzin CA, Parsons DS: Paranasal sinus bony anatomic variations and mucosal abnormalities: CT analysis for endoscopic sinus surgery. *Laryngoscope* 101:56–64, 1991.

Earwaker J: Anatomic variants in sino nasal CT. *Radiographics* 13:381–415, 1993.

Figueroa RE, Kuhn FA: Imaging evaluation for functional endoscopic sinus surgery. In Taveras J, Ferrucci R (eds): *Radiology: Diagnosis, Imaging, Intervention.* Philadelphia, JB Lippincott, 1995, Chapter 12B.

Hudgins PA: Complications of endoscopic sinus surgery: the role of the radiologist in prevention. *Radiol Clin North Am* 31:21–32, 1993.

Kuhn FA, Bolger WE, Tisdal RG: The agger nasi cell in frontal recess obstruction: anatomic, radiologic and clinical correlation. *Oper Tech Otolaryngol Head Neck Surg* 2:226–231, 1991.

Mafee MF, Chow JM, Meyers R: Functional endoscopic sinus surgery: anatomy, CT screening, indications and complications. *AJR* 160:735–744, 1993.

Ohnishi T, Tachibana T, Kaneko Y, et al: High risk areas in endoscopic sinus surgery and prevention of complications. *Laryngoscope* 103:1181–1185, 1993.

Stammberger H: Secretion transportation. In Stammberger H: *Functional Endoscopic Sinus Surgery: The Messerklinger Technique.* Philadelphia, BC Decker, 1991, pp 17–31.

Stammberger H: Special endoscopic anatomy of the lateral nasal wall and ethmoidal sinuses. In Stammberger H: *Functional Endoscopic Sinus Surgery: The Messerklinger Technique.* Philadelphia, BC Decker, 1991, pp 49–87.

Vleming M, Middelweerd RJ, de Vries N: Complications of endoscopic sinus surgery. *Arch Otol Laryngol Head Neck Surg* 118:617–623, 1992.

Zinreich SJ, Kennedy DW, Rusinbine AE: Paranasal sinuses: CT imaging requirements for endoscopic surgery. *Radiology* 163:769–775, 1987.

4

Powered Nasal Polypectomy

Joseph P. Mirante, M.D., M.B.A., F.A.C.S.
John H. Krouse, M.D., Ph.D., F.A.C.S.

The formation of focal enlargements of the nasal mucosa leads to the development of nasal polyps. This process of hypertrophic swelling can be the result of local alterations in the mucosa or from systemic disease. Although the exact pathophysiology of polyp formation has been elusive, the description of the condition and basic treatment have been part of medical practice for thousands of years.

HISTORY

Background

Early documentation in the form of a written description of nasal polyps can be traced back to Indian writings dated from 1000 B.C.[1] The treatment of polyps also has a long history. Ancient methods of polyp removal included extirpation by the use of sponges and string passed from the nose into the pharynx with a forced withdrawal. This method continued to be documented as late as the 1900s.[2] The treatment of polyps was also done with cautery or caustic solutions as early as the time of Hippocrates.[3] From the time of Galen, nasal polyps were thought to be a manifestation of systemic disease occurring from a thickening of the body's humors. Galen's significant experience with surgical procedures included removal of nasal polyps.[4]

The rise of European civilization with eventual spread to the new world saw little change in the basic treatment of nasal polyps except for alteration in tools reflecting the current technology. In the Middle Ages, knotted strings were used as saws to remove polyps.[2] In the 1500s a method of removal employed the use of harpsichord wire and a tube, and, by the turn of the next century removal of polyps utilizing forceps was discovered.[2]

Throughout the 1700s advances were made in rhinology including the use of drainage procedures with stenting and the development of approaches to the maxillary and frontal sinuses. Continued advancement of concepts of anatomy, histology, and pathophysiology allowed for better understanding of disease processes. The idea of nasal polyps as a local phenomena resulting from sinonasal disease was introduced in the 1700s.[3] This was later confirmed by Billroth in the next century who was of the opinion that polyps were an adenomatous formation.

The historic treatment of nasal polyps, caustics, cautery, and gross removal have continued essentially unchanged into the twentieth century, albeit with modern technical additions such as electric cautery and the use of snares or forceps. Theories of polyp formation, however, have undergone a constant and more significant evolution.

Incidence

The exact incidence of nasal polyposis in the general population has not been determined. There have been studies, however, in smaller populations more at risk due to systemic disease or those with atopy. Systemic conditions associated with polyp formation include bronchial asthma, cystic fibrosis, Young's syndrome, or Kartagener's syndrome.

Aspirin intolerance has been closely linked with polyp formation and the important clinical association of the triad of aspirin sensitivity, asthma, and nasal polyps has been greatly described.

A 1995 review noted an incidence of nasal polyps of 0.5% in atopic patients.[5] In cystic fibrosis the incidence is approximately 20%. Nasal polyps have been reported in as high as 36% of cases with asthmatic patients who are aspirin sensitive.[1]

Pathology

Grossly, nasal polyps are the formation of edematous tissue and present as a smooth soft lesion that can be clear, yellow, or reddish in color (Figure 4.1). Polyp size is variable, and they often present bilaterally (Figure 4.2). Polyps tend to arise from a stalk and are insensate. Histologically polyps consist of respiratory epithelium surrounding an exceedingly inflammatory stroma. There is a noticeable absence of the secretory glands found in normal respiratory epithelium and a significant influx of inflammatory cells with a predominance of eosinophils.[5]

Pathophysiology

The exact series of histologic events that lead to the formation of nasal polyps remains uncertain. Several key factors appear to be instrumental in their development including chronic infection, vasomotor responses, and the ensuing mucosa edema. Multiple pathogenic models have been proposed based on deductions from these findings along with the histologic changes.

Polyp formation as a type of neoplasia was proposed in earlier theories such as Billroth's adenoma formation in 1855 or Hopman's fibroma theory in 1885.[6] The neoplastic theories were later discounted as were the mechanical theories of polyp formation. In these discussions it was postulated that the progressive enlargement of subepithelial tissues occurred through persistent edema, increased laxity, and subsequent expansion into the nasal cavity as polyps.[1]

Theories of polyp formation through vasomotor effects on vascular permeability with subsequent

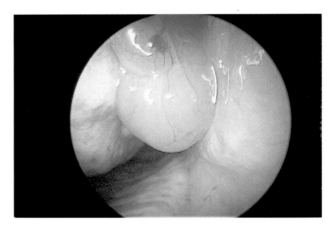

Figure 4.1. Endoscopic view of a nasal polyp.

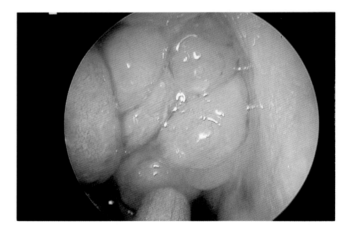

Figure 4.2. Multilobular nasal polyp.

increases in submucosal edema or through inflammatory infiltrates expanding submucosal edema have also been proposed. These discussions support the formation of a local process but have not clearly made the link from the occurrence of edema to polyp formation. Additional current theories have explored the role of infection and have targeted immunologic processes, particularly mediated through IgE, to explain the process.

The role of infection in polyp formation has also been uncertain. Infection clearly plays a secondary role in patients with polyps due to obstruction of sinus ostia and subsequent stasis. A primary role for infection has generated more debate. An experimental study by Norlander used a rabbit model to simulate purulent sinusitis by creating obstruction of the maxillary sinuses and introducing various bacteria. The formation of polyps after infection was independent of the specific bacterial agent and damage to the nasal mucosa was concluded to be of greatest importance in polyp formation.[7] The potential of bacteria to cause epithelial damage appeared to be the necessary factor for polyp formation.

Currently research has focused on the immunologic aspects of polyp formation to explain the etiology. The presence of specific inflammatory cell populations has been well associated with polyp formation. Histologic examination of polypoid stroma has shown evidence of degranulating mast cells, the presence of active chemical mediators of the inflammatory process, and the presence of allergen-specific IgE. The correlation of nasal polyps and allergy has also supported this line of investigation.[1] Technical advances in immunology and molecular biology have taken the investigation of the process down to the molecular level in an attempt to tie these factors into a cogent theory of polyp formation.

Powered Instrumentation

Interest in powered dissection techniques in otolaryngology dates back to the late 1960s, when Urban developed a vacuum rotary device for use in acoustic neuroma surgery.[8] In the past 5 years this type of instrument has been popularized for use in nasal and sinus surgery. Through the adaptation of orthopedic "soft tissue shavers," several surgeons began to utilize this technology for the removal of polyps and other soft tissue masses in the nasal cavity. In an early paper Hawke and McCombe[13] describe the use of one such device in a series of 50 patients with nasal polyps who underwent surgery in an office setting. The authors reported excellent results through the use of this method, and reported that nasal packing was unnecessary in this sample.

Other authors described the use of microdebriders in the operating room setting for both the removal of soft and bony tissues. Setliff[9] reported his experience with 345 patients, many of whom had significant nasal polypoid disease. In addition, Christmas and Krouse[10] reported excellent results in the treatment of extensive sinonasal polyposis through a powered dissection technique. Outcome data regarding this approach were also reported by these authors, demonstrating the safety and efficacy of the powered technique.[11]

Additionally, Krouse and Christmas[12] report on the use of an office-based approach to nasal polyp disease utilizing the microdebrider. They note that patients can be operated upon quite easily and comfortably with this technique. As reported by Hawke and McCombe,[13] nasal packing was not necessary, and bleeding was minimal in this group of patients. Furthermore, Gross and Becker[14] have reported that the microdebrider has particular usefulness in the treatment of severe nasal polyposis.

Early experience with powered instrumentation in nasal polyp surgery has shown it to be easy to perform, relatively bloodless, and quite safe and effective. The technique can be used as part of an extensive hospital-based approach to severe sinonasal polyposis, but also has utility for limited disease in the office setting where extensive sinus surgery is not indicated. The ability of the powered devices to easily remove soft tissue from the nasal cavity makes them ideal instruments for the surgical treatment of nasal polyposis.

SURGICAL TECHNIQUE

Hemostasis and Anesthesia

As with any nasal and sinus surgical procedure, meticulous hemostasis is important in allowing a safe and comfortable operating field. Whether the procedure is performed under local or general anesthesia, or within a hospital or office setting, the patient first sprays the nose with oxymetazoline 0.05% 15 to 20 min prior to beginning the surgical procedure. The use of this topical decongestant begins the process of vasoconstriction. The patient is then brought to the surgical suite or treatment room where anesthesia is induced.

When general anesthesia is utilized, induction is performed at this point. With the patient asleep in the operating room, the nose is then packed with cotton pledgets impregnated with 1:1,000 epinephrine. In our experience the use of this concentration of epinephrine has never provoked any untoward reactions. The pledgets are placed in the nose adjacent to the polypoid tissue. Pledgets are left in position for 10 min and then removed. The polypoid tissue itself is then injected with 1% xylocaine with 1:100,000 epinephrine. As the tissue is removed, additional injections or sequential use of epinephrine-impregnated cotton can be useful in achieving vasoconstriction more posteriorly in the nasal cavity.

In the office setting, with the patient seated comfortably in the exam chair (Figure 4.3), the nose is next sprayed with tetracaine 2% and with a vasoconstricting agent such as ephedrine 3%. Cotton pledgets impregnated with a mixture of these two agents can then be placed into the nose and left in position for 10 to 15 min. Injection of the polypoid tissue is then performed using xylocaine 1% with

epinephrine 1:100,000 (Figure 4.4). As dissection of the polypoid tissue proceeds, additional topical anesthetic use is often necessary. In addition, in the office setting supplement anesthesia can be of utility. Depending on the surgeon's preferences, and the extent of the disease to be removed, injections can be made into the lateral nasal wall, the inferior and middle turbinates, and the region of the infraorbital nerve. In addition, sphenopalatine block transorally can be performed, but the potential complications associated with this technique must be considered. Injection of the nasal septum is usually not necessary, and often results in troublesome bleeding during the procedure.

Surgical Technique

Polypoid disease in the nose is especially amenable to the use of the powered microdebrider due to its texture and pedunculated nature. Adequate suction pressure is necessary, but for the removal of polypoid disease is not required to be as strong as in more extensive surgery of the sinuses. The routine treatment cabinet available in otolaryngology offices provides sufficient suction for effective removal of

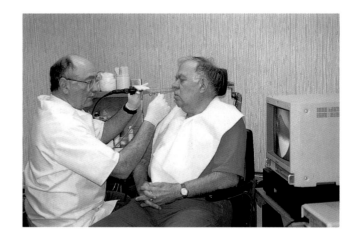

Figure 4.3. Positioning of the patient for office nasal polypectomy.

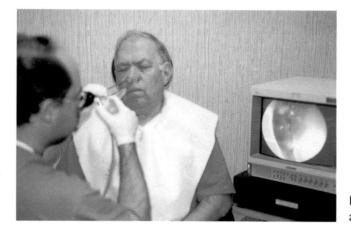

Figure 4.4. Intranasal injection of local anesthesia.

polypoid disease in most cases. The surgeon approximates the cutting port of the device to the free edge of the polypoid tissue, allowing the tissue to be drawn into the port by the suction pressure (Figures 4.5 and 4.6). The device is then actuated with the footpedal, allowing the polyps to be sheared off and suctioned out. The console of the microdebrider is set in the oscillating mode to allow efficient removal

of tissue without blockage of the device. Dissection proceeds posterosuperiorly and the polypoid tissue traced to its origin. In-office polypectomy dissection is completed when all visible polypoid tissue is removed from the nose. If sinus surgery is to be performed in combination with this polypectomy, dissection will continue as described elsewhere in this text.

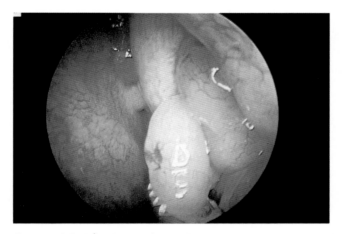

Figure 4.5. Nasal polyp being drawn into open cannula of the microdebrider.

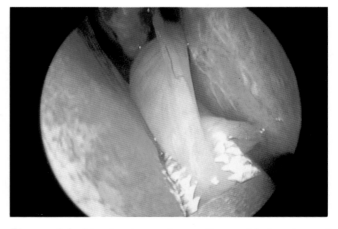

Figure 4.6. Nasal polyp under suction and being sheared off as drawn into the microdebrider.

Through the use of the microdebrider technique bleeding is less than with avulsive methods in nasal and sinus surgery. Nasal packing, therefore, is rarely necessary, even when extensive resection is performed. In addition, the use of systemic corticosteroid treatment preoperatively has not been necessary, and is not routinely utilized.

CONCLUSION

The use of powered dissection in the performance of nasal polypectomies has been a safe and effective method and has been adopted by a number of otolaryngologists. It is easily learned, and can be performed without difficulty even by less experienced surgeons. Since many surgeons are just now beginning to adopt this technique in their sinus surgery, they may feel more comfortable in the use of powered dissection of polypoid disease as a first step in the acquisition of these skills. With increasing experience, their move into more bony work can therefore be facilitated.

REFERENCES

1. Frenkiel S, Small P: Pathogenesis and treatment of nasal polyps. In Blitzer A, Lawson W, Freideman W (eds): *Surgery of the Paranasal Sinuses.* Philadelphia, WB Saunders, 1991.
2. McFarland GE: A brief history of otolaryngology. *J Am Acad Ophth Otol* 78:15–20, 1974.
3. Leopold D: A history of rhinology in North America. *Otolaryngol Head Neck Surg* 115: 283–297, 1996.
4. Haeger K: *The Illustrated History of Surgery.* Gottenburg, Bell, 1988.
5. Bernstein JM, Gorfein J, Noble B: Role of allergy in nasal polyposis: a review. *Otolaryngol Head Neck Surg* 113:724–732, 1995.
6. Tos M: The pathogenic theories on formation of nasal polyps. *Am J Rhinol* 4:51–56, 1990.
7. Norlander T, Fukami M, Westrin KM, et al: Formation of mucosal polyps in the nasal and maxillary sinus cavities by infection. *Otolaryngol Head Neck Surg* 109:522–529, 1993.
8. House WF, Hitselberger WE: Surgical complications of acoustic tumor surgery. *Arch Otolaryngol* 88:659–667, 1968.
9. Setliff RC, Parsons DS. The "Hummer": new instrumentation for functional endoscopic sinus surgery. *Am J Rhinol* 8:275–278, 1994.
10. Christmas DA, Krouse JH: Powered instrumentation in functional endoscopic sinus surgery I: surgical technique. *Ear Nose Throat J* 75:33–40, 1996.
11. Krouse JH, Christmas DA: Powered instrumentation in functional endoscopic sinus surgery II: a comparative study. *Ear Nose Throat J* 75:42–44, 1996.
12. Krouse JH, Christmas DA: Powered nasal polypectomy in the office setting. *Ear Nose Throat J* 75:608–610, 1996.
13. Hawke WM, McCombe AW: How I do it: nasal polypectomy with an arthroscopic bone shaver: the Stryker "Hummer." *J Otolaryngol* 24:57–59, 1995.
14. Gross CW, Becker DG: Power instrumentation in endoscopic sinus surgery. *Oper Tech Otolaryngol Head Neck Surgery.* 7:236–241, 1996.

5

Powered Dissection of the Ethmoid Sinuses

Dewey A. Christmas, Jr., M.D.
John H. Krouse, M.D., Ph.D., F.A.C.S.

BACKGROUND

Traditionally, ethmoid sinus surgery was late to develop due to the relative danger of the technique. In fact, Mosher commented in 1929 that ". . . it [ethmoid sinus surgery] has proved to be one of the easiest operations with which to kill a patient."[1(p870)] The first ethmoid procedures were performed via the transantral route, as otolaryngologists gained comfort with maxillary sinus surgery. In this procedure, as originally described by Jansen,[2] both the inferior and middle turbinates were removed, along with the entire lateral nasal wall. As a result, atrophic rhinitis and its inherent symptoms was the common consequence, leading to a decrease in the popularity of the approach.

In 1912 Mosher first published his description of an intranasal approach to ethmoidectomy.[3] While many physicians were successful in the application of the technique, it was quite a dangerous operation, and many serious surgical complications occurred. The intranasal ethmoidectomy therefore became used much less frequently, and approaches to the ethmoid sinuses were done via external incisions under direct visualization over the next 50 years. With the development of endoscopic devices which allowed direct and accurate visualization of the anatomy of the nose, intranasal ethmoidectomy again increased in popularity in the 1980s.[4,5]

Since 1985, functional endoscopic surgery has become the primary approach to the paranasal sinuses. Kennedy introduced this technique to American otolaryngologists at that time, allowing a more precise method of sinus surgery accompanied by a significant decrease in complications.

ANATOMY AND PHYSIOLOGY

Of all the paranasal sinuses, the ethmoid system has the greatest variability. In the adult, the ethmoid sinuses form a pyramid, with the wider base at the posterior aspect of the ethmoid system. In anteroposterior dimension the ethmoid sinuses measure 4 to 5 cm. The sinuses average 2.5 cm in height, and 0.5 to 1.5 cm in width.[1] The roof of the sinus, known as the *fovea ethmoidalis*, extends superiorly to the more medial cribriform plate. The medial aspect of the fovea is especially vulnerable to injury and is the most frequent site of intracranial entry in sinus surgery due to its relative thinness compared to the surrounding bone. At times the height of this fovea can be exaggerated, leading to prominent olfactory grooves, and an increased susceptibility to injury.[6]

The ethmoid system is best appreciated as a labyrinth containing a variable number of cells. Van Alyea[8] reported an average of 9 cells per side, with a range of 4 to 17 cells in a cadaver study. This variability confirms the intricacies involved in surgical approaches to this area. The anteriormost cells of the ethmoid system form an area referred to as the *frontal recess*, the area in which the frontal sinus empties into the nasal cavity. This frontal recess can be considered as an inverted funnel bounded laterally by the lateral nasal wall, medially by the middle turbinate, posteriorly and superiorly by the skull base, and anteriorly by the agger nasi cell.[7] The agger nasi is the most constant of the cells and is formed by pneumatization of the lacrimal bone.[8]

As the middle turbinate is gently reflected, the next of the major ethmoid structures is encountered, the *bulla ethmoidalis.* This prominence is a reliable surgical landmark and is a consistent anatomic structure. The anterior ethmoid cells are then located just posterior to the anterior face of the bulla. Continuing posteriorly, the *basal lamella* or *ground lamella* of the middle turbinate is encountered. This structure separates the anterior ethmoid cells from the posterior ethmoid cells. The posterior boundary of the ethmoid sinuses is encountered at the anterior face of the sphenoid sinus. Disease in these ethmoid cells is felt to be the key to chronic disease in the maxillary and frontal sinuses.

A common anatomic variant which is encountered in many patients is the *Onodi cell.* This cell is actually a large pneumatized posterior ethmoid cell, which pneumatizes lateral and superior to the sphenoid sinus. This structure is of importance in surgical approaches to the ethmoid, since the optic nerve frequently makes an impression on the lateral wall of the Onodi cell. The optic nerve is especially sensitive to injury in this area, and in fact more cases of optic nerve injury are encountered in the posterior ethmoid than in the sphenoid sinus.

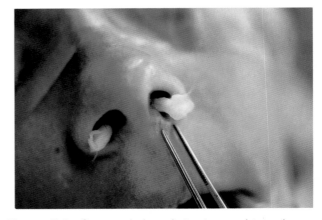

Figure 5.1. Cotton pledgets being inserted into the nasal airways.

The hemostatic procedure begins prior to the patient entering the operating room. While the patient is in the operative holding area, he or she sprays the nose bilaterally with 0.05% oxymetazoline spray 15 to 20 min before coming to the operating suite. After general anesthesia is induced, or prior to infiltration of local anesthetic agents, cotton pledgets (Figure 5.1) with 1:1,000 epinephrine (Figure 5.2) are inserted along the inferior and middle turbinates. These pledgets are left in position for 10 min to provide decongestion of the mucosa of the nose.

SURGICAL APPROACHES

Hemostasis

In all methods of sinus surgery, safe technique requires a bloodless field. Not only is bleeding dangerous as it obscures the landmarks necessary to complete a safe operation, but it is also frustrating for the surgeon who is attempting to perform a successful procedure. Time spent in achieving excellent hemostasis will reduce operating time during the dissection, and will provide a relatively clean field, obviating the need for nasal packing postoperatively. Packing is often the major source of discomfort and morbidity in the immediate postoperative period.

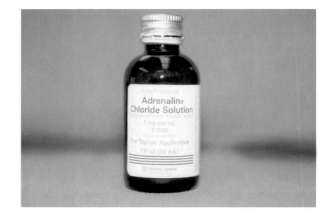

Figure 5.2. Topical epinephrine solution, 1:1,000.

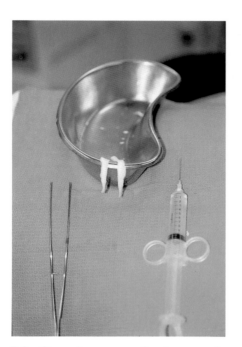

Figure 5.3. Operative set-up for hemostasis and local anesthesia.

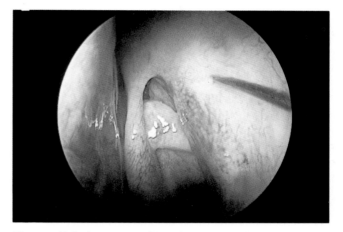

Figure 5.4. Injection of local anesthetic/vasoconstrictor near the insertion of the middle turbinate into the lateral nasal wall.

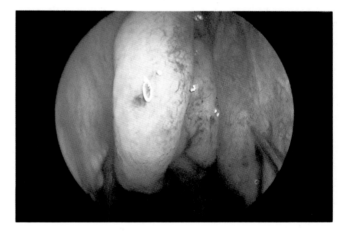

Figure 5.5. Injection at the junction of the uncinate process and the lateral nasal wall.

At this point, injection of 1% xylocaine with 1:100,000 epinephrine (Figure 5.3) is made into the nasal membranes. A submucosal injection is carried out starting superiorly just above the insertion of the middle turbinate with the lateral wall of the nose (Figure 5.4). A blanching can be visualized with the endoscope as the injection is performed. Further injections are performed proceeding inferiorly along the lateral nasal wall, at the junction of the insertion of the uncinate process with the lateral wall of the nose (Figure 5.5). Blanching will be noted of the lateral nasal wall and of the uncinate process with this injection. It is also important to inject the anterior surface of the middle turbinate (Figure 5.6) so that any manipulation of this structure does not result in annoying bleeding during the remainder of the procedure. An additional injection is made at the inferior insertion of the uncinate process posteriorly and over the face of the ethmoid bulla (Figure 5.7). A supplemental injection can then be made in the region of the sphenopalatine artery at its entrance to the nose. This area corresponds to the junction of the posterior wall of the maxillary sinus with the lateral nasal wall (Figure 5.8). This final injection provides excellent control of bleeding attributable to the branches of the sphenopalatine artery. It is as effective as an intraoral injection of the sphenopalatine canal, and does not carry with it the potential

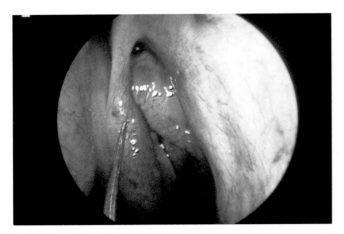

Figure 5.6. Injection into the anterior surface of the middle turbinate.

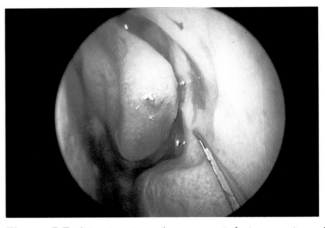

Figure 5.7. Injection into the posteroinferior portion of the uncinate process and over the face of the ethmoid bulla.

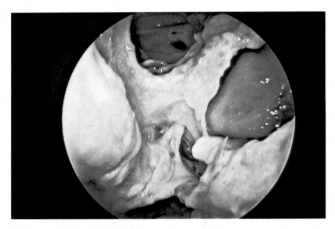

Figure 5.8. Exit of the sphenopalatine artery into the nasal cavity.

for serious complications noted with the latter procedure. Once the nasal membranes have been sufficiently decongested, the cotton pledgets with epinephrine can be inserted into the middle meatus and left in place until the beginning of the surgical procedure. The use of cocaine hydrochloride is not necessary in this approach to hemostasis.

Uncinectomy

Identification of the uncinate process is first made by gently displacing the middle turbinate medially, being careful not to fracture its attachment superiorly. This maneuver can be accomplished with a Freer elevator or with a double balled-probe or Lusk seeker (Figure 5.9). The location of the uncinate process is often much more posterior than the surgeon would anticipate, and its free edge must first be identified to establish accurate anatomic localization. The free edge is then tented anteriorly by gentle pressure with a ball probe (Figure 5.10). The entire superior to inferior extent of this free edge must be confirmed in order to establish the limits of the dissection and to identify the infundibulum. It is particularly important to identify the superior insertion of the uncinate process as this area forms part of the boundary of the frontal recess.

It is first necessary to achieve a rough edge in the uncinate process for the microdebrider to purchase. The method in which the instrument functions requires this rough surface in order to allow the rotating blade to grasp a bit of tissue and draw it into the inner cannula for dissection. Sufficient suction is critical in the adequate functioning of the microdebrider, and a frequent source of frustration and difficulty in dissection is poor suction pressure

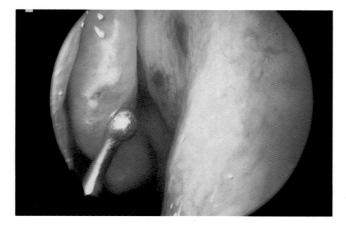

Figure 5.9. Ball probe displacing the middle turbinate.

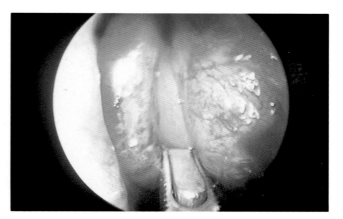

Figure 5.11. Side biting pediatric forceps in the middle meatus.

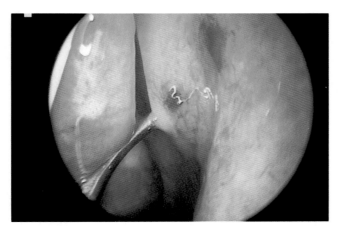

Figure 5.10. Ball probe behind free edge of the uncinate process.

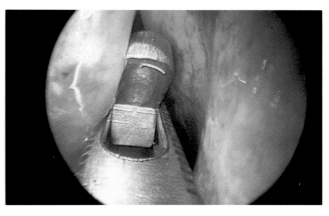

Figure 5.12. Side biting forceps placed posterior to the uncinate edge with the cutting blade opened.

delivered to the handpiece. To create this edge in the uncinate process, a window of tissue is removed using a side-biting forceps (Figure 5.11). The opening of the forceps is placed posterior to the uncinate process and the cutting blade is opened (Figure 5.12) and located so as to grasp the uncinate process in a posterior to anterior orientation (Figure 5.13).

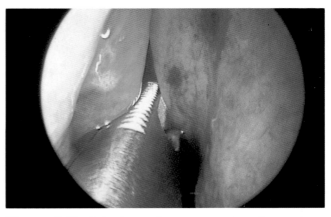

Figure 5.13. Side biting forceps grasping the uncinate process in a posterior to anterior orientation.

Several small bites are taken through the uncinate process in a medial to lateral direction to create a small window (Figures 5.14–5.16). An alternate approach to creating this window involves the use of the ball probe (Figures 5.17–5.19). The probe can also serve as a tearing device, creating a rent transversely from the insertion of the uncinate process to the free edge medially. Either of the above methods will create a sufficient surface for the microdebrider to grasp, thereby allowing a safe and effective surgical procedure.

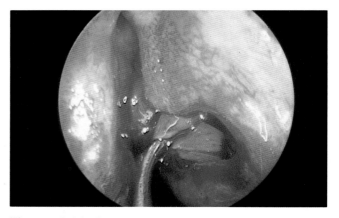

Figure 5.16. Small window created in the uncinate process.

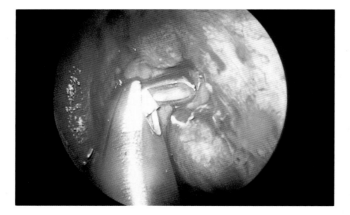

Figure 5.14. Small window created in the uncinate process.

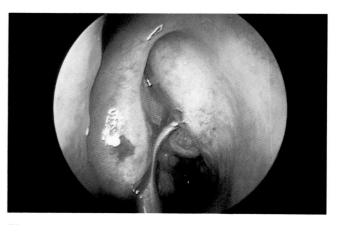

Figure 5.17. Alternate approach to creating an uncinate window using a ball probe.

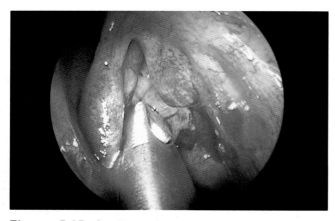

Figure 5.15. Small window created in the uncinate process.

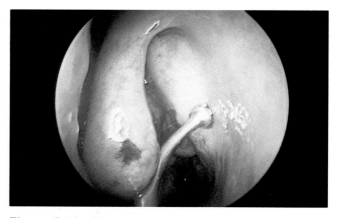

Figure 5.18. Alternate approach to creating an uncinate window using a ball probe.

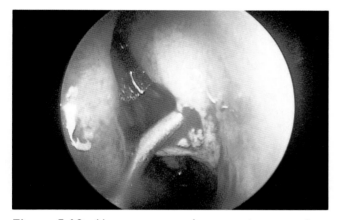

Figure 5.19. Alternate approach to creating an uncinate window using a ball probe.

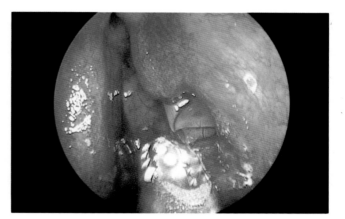

Figure 5.20. Uncinectomy.

The uncinate process can then be removed using the microdebrider from the inferior attachment of the uncinate to its superior insertion in the frontal recess (Figures 5.20–5.22). The 4-mm serrated bits are preferred for dissection of the ethmoid system. A gentle wiping or rolling motion of the microdebrider tip is used (Figures 5.23–5.25). This technique allows tissue to be drawn into the device and transected by the rotating shaft. It is important to stress that pressure is not necessary in the removal of the tissue; rather, allowing the tissue to be drawn into the suction and sheared off provides the proper method for dissection. In the dissection of the inferior portion of the uncinate process, it is very important to remove this entire area of tissue (Figure 5.26). Lateral to this inferior uncinate is the natural ostium of the maxillary sinus (Figure 5.27), and tissue allowed to remain in this location is a major source of recurrent or persistent sinusitis. At the conclusion of the dissection of the uncinate process (Figure 5.28), the edges of the mucosa are seamed together so that little exposed bone is present, obviating the need for extensive reepithelialization.

Ethmoid Sinusotomy

The approach to the ethmoid sinus can be carried out in one of two ways. The more conventional approach to the ethmoid involves dissection through the anterior wall of the ethmoid bulla (Figure 5.29).

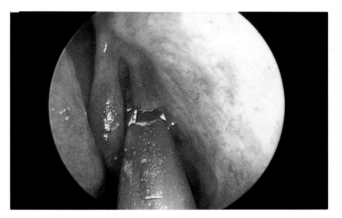

Figure 5.21. Uncinectomy.

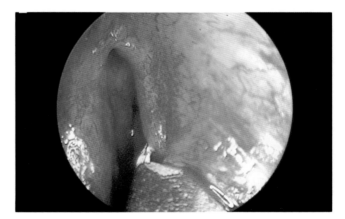

Figure 5.22. Uncinectomy.

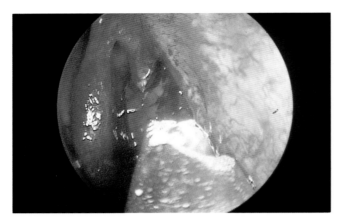

Figure 5.23. Rolling motion of the microdebrider.

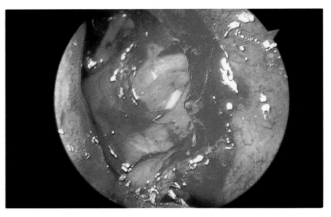

Figure 5.26. Inferior remnant of the uncinate process.

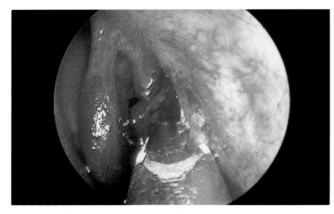

Figure 5.24. Rolling motion of the microdebrider.

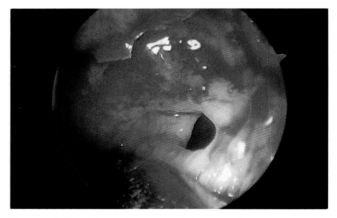

Figure 5.27. Natural ostium of the maxillary sinus.

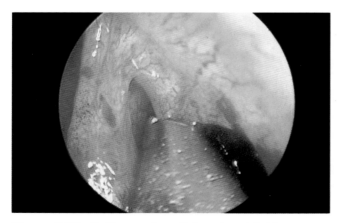

Figure 5.25. Rolling motion of the microdebrider.

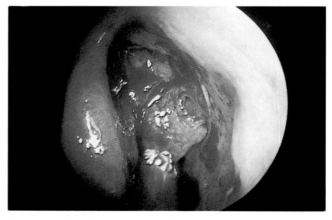

Figure 5.28. Completed uncinectomy.

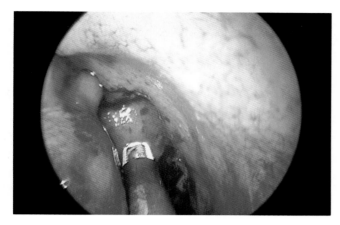

Figure 5.29. Anterior wall of the ethmoid bulla.

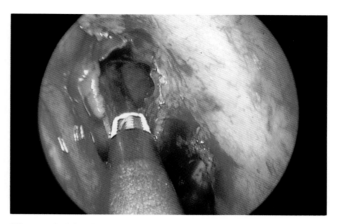

Figure 5.31. Enlargement of the opening into the ethmoid bulla using a rolling motion.

The microdebrider bit is inserted through the thin bone of the anterior face of the bulla ethmoidalis (Figure 5.30). A gentle circumferential dissection is then performed from the center area where the microdebrider perforated the bulla outward using a rolling motion of the microdebrider (Figures 5.31 and 5.32). A second technique involves approaching the bulla ethmoidalis from medial to lateral. In this method, dissection is carried from the safety of the medial ethmoid toward the lamina papyracea laterally. Again a gentle rolling motion is used, allowing the tissue to be drawn into the microdebrider. It is important to preserve both the superior attachment

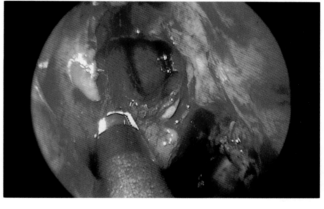

Figure 5.32. Enlargement of the opening into the ethmoid bulla using a rolling motion.

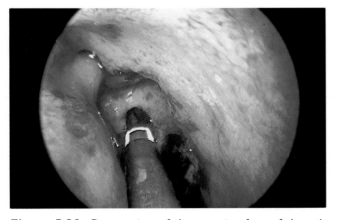

Figure 5.30. Penetration of the anterior face of the ethmoid bulla.

of the middle turbinate and the inferiormost axial strut of the bulla ethmoidalis (Figure 5.33) in order to lessen the likelihood of lateralization of the middle turbinate and its consequences. As dissection is taken posteriorly, the anterior ethmoid cells are systematically exenterated in a rolling method.

After the anterior ethmoid dissection is completed, the ground lamella is penetrated with the microdebrider (Figure 5.34), and the opening enlarged circumferentially (Figure 5.35). Dissection continues into the posterior ethmoid system (Figure 5.36), again relying upon this rolling technique.

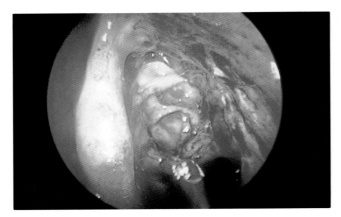

Figure 5.33. Preservation of the transverse axial strut of the ethmoid bulla.

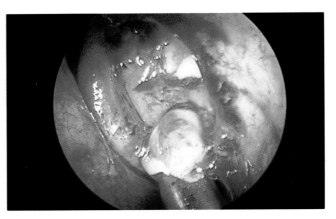

Figure 5.36. Continuation of the dissection into the posterior ethmoid cells.

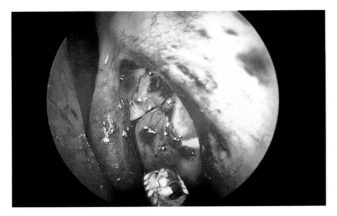

Figure 5.34. Penetration of the ground lamella with the microdebrider.

Throughout the dissection, remember that the weakest point of the ethmoid roof is medially, where the bone is thinnest near the cribriform lamella. Penetration of the skull base is easiest in this area (Figure 5.37).[9] As the posterior ethmoid is approached, it must be remembered that the ethmoid often is extensively pneumatized laterally and superiorly. A large posterior ethmoid cell is commonly encountered at this level, the so-called Onodi cell. This anatomic structure is critical to appreciate, in that the optic nerve often passes laterally through this cell and can be easily damaged with lateral dissection in this area.

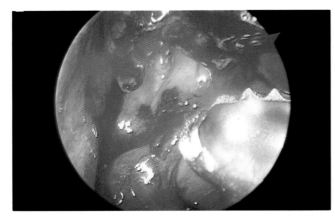

Figure 5.35. Circumferential enlargement into the opening of the ground lamella.

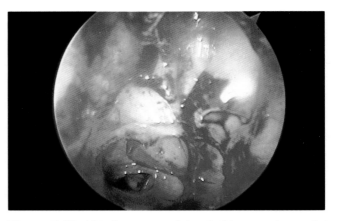

Figure 5.37. Weak portion of the skull base in the medial ethmoid cells.

It is important to remember that this operation is a functional procedure and not a cosmetic dissection. The microdebrider can be used parallel to the skull base safely and need not be used to remove every remnant of ethmoid cell walls along the skull base (Figure 5.38). The purpose of the procedure is to exteriorize the ethmoid system in order to improve ventilation and drainage. This result can be achieved without dissecting the skull base to a smooth polished plate of bone.

Use of the microdebrider for ethmoidectomy offers several advantages. First, the integral suction in the powered device allows small amounts of blood often encountered during the surgery to be easily cleared without having to stop the procedure and use a separate suction. Surgery can therefore continue without the frequent need to change instruments within the operating field. In addition, dissection is carried out with the microdebrider in a plane parallel to the skull base and lamina papyracea, thereby increasing the safety of the procedure. The circumferential rolling motion used to dissect the ethmoid system allows for a safe and effective removal of diseased tissue, as well as preserving the normal mucosa and preventing aggressive deepithelialization of this mucosa (Figures 5.39 and 5.40).

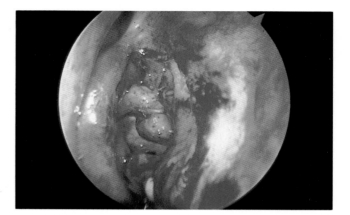

Figure 5.39. Completion of the ethmoid dissection.

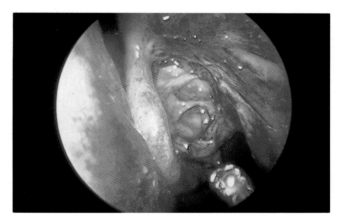

Figure 5.40. Completion of the ethmoid dissection.

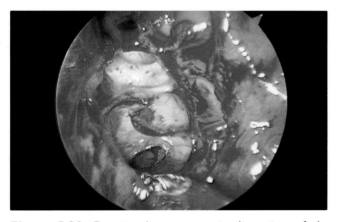

Figure 5.38. Functional, noncosmetic dissection of the skull base.

Concha Bullosa Resection

In cases in which a large, extensively pneumatized middle turbinate creates a significant obstruction to the osteomeatal unit (Figure 5.41), the microdebrider provides an excellent tool for reshaping this anatomic abnormality and reestablishing normal aeration and drainage. The concha bullosa can be entered anteriorly by punching through with the microdebrider bit, much as is done in entering the bulla ethmoidalis (Figure 5.42). The opening is enlarged circumferentially (Figure 5.43), and the lateral aspect of the concha bullosa is then removed posterior to the level of the free edge of the uncinate

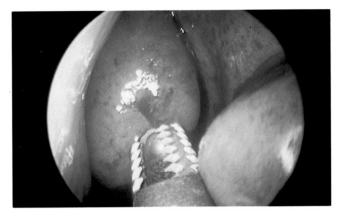

Figure 5.41. Large concha bullosa of the middle turbinate obstructing the osteomeatal complex.

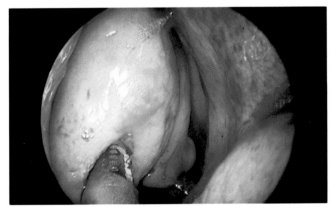

Figure 5.42. Microdebrider entering the anterior face of the concha bullosa.

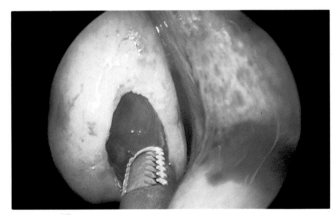

Figure 5.43. Circumferential enlargement of the opening into the anterior face of the concha bullosa.

process (Figure 5.44) through the use of the microdebrider (Figure 5.45). The medial portion of the middle turbinate is therefore maintained (Figure 5.46). This procedure is easy to perform and quite safe, and opens up the previously narrowed middle meatus quite well, reestablishing more normal function.

The microdebrider can also be used to thin or trim large bulky middle turbinates which are not pneumatized in order to open the middle meatus adequately. In addition, when floppy middle turbinates are encountered, either as a result of the surgical technique or from polypoid disease, they can easily be trimmed or reshaped in order to prevent lateralization and reocclusion of the middle meatus.

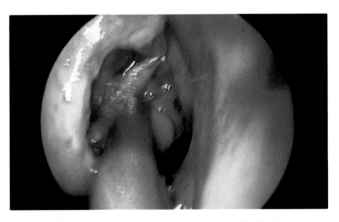

Figure 5.44. Removal of the lateral wall of the concha bullosa posterior to the free edge of the uncinate process.

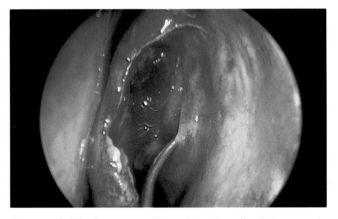

Figure 5.45. Removal of the lateral wall of the concha bullosa posterior to the free edge of the uncinate process.

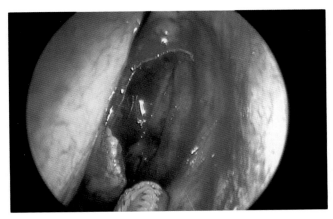

Figure 5.46. Completion of the resection, with the medial portion of the concha bullosa maintained.

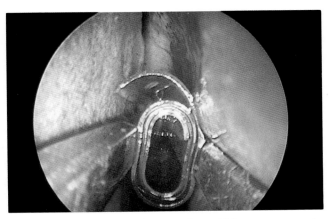

Figure 5.47. Gelfilm splints in the middle meatus at the conclusion of the ethmoid dissection.

Conclusion of the Surgery

The use of electrocautery has rarely been necessary in dissection of the ethmoid sinuses. It can be of some benefit in lightly cauterizing the free edge of a concha bullosa resection posteriorly if the surgeon feels it is necessary. The nose is not packed after the procedure, decreasing patient discomfort during the immediate postoperative recovery period. At the conclusion of the case, rolled Gelfilm splints are placed into the middle meatus in order to stent the area between the middle turbinate and the lateral nasal wall (Figure 5.47). These splints are left in position for 1 to 2 weeks, and if they have not extruded spontaneously at that time are removed in the office under endoscopic visualization.

REFERENCES

1. Mosher HP: The surgical anatomy of the ethmoid labyrinth. *Ann Otol Rhinol Laryngol* 38:869–890, 1929.
2. Jansen A: Die Killian'sche Radical-Operation Chronischer Stirnhohleneiterungen. *Ohren Nasen Kehlkopfheil* 56:110–112, 1902.
3. Mosher HP: The applied anatomy and the intranasal surgery of the ethmoid labyrinth. *Trans Am Laryngol Assoc* 34:25–45, 1912.
4. Kennedy DW: Functional endoscopic sinus surgery. *Arch Otolaryngol* 111:643–649, 1985.
5. Stammberger H: Endoscopic endonasal surgery—concepts in treatment of recurring rhinosinusitis. *Otolaryngol Head Neck Surg* 94:143–156, 1986.
6. Rice DH, Schaefer SD: *Endoscopic Paranasal Sinus Surgery,* ed 2. New York, Raven Press, 1993.
7. Kuhn FA, Bolger WE, Tisdal, RG: The agger nasi cell in frontal recess obstruction: an anatomic, radiologic and clinical correlation. *Oper Tech Otolaryngol Head Neck Surg* 2:226–231, 1991.
8. Van Alyea OE: Ethmoid labyrinth. Anatomic study, with consideration of the clinical significance of its structural characteristics. *Arch Otolaryngol* 29:881–902, 1939.
9. Kainz J, Stammberger H: The roof of the anterior ethmoid: a place of least resistance in the skull base. *Am J Rhinol* 3:191–200, 1989.

6

Powered Dissection of the Maxillary Sinus

Dewey A. Christmas, Jr., M.D.
John H. Krouse, M.D., Ph.D., F.A.C.S.

BACKGROUND

Approaches to the maxillary sinus have been quite variable over the past century. During the late nineteenth century, an understanding of the anatomy of the maxillary sinus led to a philosophy of drainage of the maxillary antrum as the primary treatment for infection in the paranasal sinuses. Early surgeons felt that drainage of this empyema could best be accomplished through the most dependent location, often involving the removal of a molar tooth and drainage directly into the mouth.[1] While drainage was facilitated in this manner, cures of the underlying pathology were rare due to what we now realize is inadequate ventilation and restoration of normal physiologic function.

Maxillary sinus surgery became commonly performed through the work of two surgeons in the late 1800s. George Caldwell,[2] practicing in New York, and Henri Luc[3] of France independently developed a radical antrostomy procedure in which a trephination into the anterior face of the maxillary antrum was widened and the sinus cavity approached through this incision with removal of bone. In addition, aeration of the sinus was established, with inferior antrostomy by Caldwell and middle meatal antrostomy by Luc. In this procedure, mucosa was stripped radically from the cavity, resulting in regrowth of abnormal mucosa with less efficient ciliary function, as well as replacement of much of this mucosa with dense fibrotic material. The so-called "Caldwell–Luc"[4] procedure was widely performed until the 1980s. While still a common procedure, it has been done less often since the advent of endoscopic techniques and with the understanding of the normal physiology of the maxillary sinus and ostiomeatal complex gained in the past two decades.

While Luc advocated a middle meatal antrostomy, with the thinking that enlargement of the natural ostium of the maxillary sinus would provide the most appropriate ventilation and drainage, research done by Anderson Hilding in the late 1930s[5,6] suggested that disturbance of the maxillary ostium led to increased problems with maxillary sinus function, and that inferior antrostomies were therefore preferred for ventilation. In addition, logic suggested further that dependent drainage should be superior to procedures done in the middle meatus. Inferior antrostomy therefore became the accepted ventilation technique in maxillary sinus surgery. With an understanding of the normal physiology appreciated through the work of Messerklinger[7] and Wigand,[8] it became apparent that the mucociliary flow patterns were genetically programmed to beat toward the natural ostium in the middle meatus (Figure 6.1). Inferior antrostomy, therefore, could not be effective as it did not allow for a re-creation of the normal flow pattern. Endoscopic techniques have therefore universally established middle meatal antrostomy as the physiologically appropriate procedure.[9] With the precision afforded by these techniques it can be performed safely and effectively.

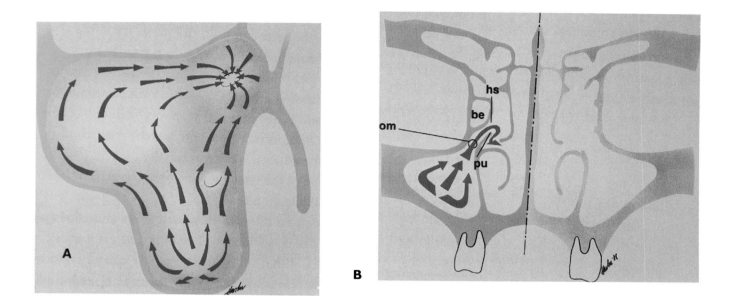

Figure 6.1. Schematic drawing of secretion transport out of a right maxillary sinus. pu = uncinate process; hs = hiatus semilunaris; be = bulla ethmoidalis; om = maxillary ostium. (From Stammberger H: *Functional Endoscopic Sinus Surgery: The Messerklinger Technique*. Philadelphia, Decker, 1991. Reprinted with permission.)

ANATOMY AND PHYSIOLOGY

The maxillary sinus is an irregularly shaped cavity, roughly resembling an inverted pyramid in an adult, and measuring about 3 cm in width, depth, and height.[10] The primary ostium (natural ostium) is located in the superior aspect of the medial wall of the maxillary sinus (Figure 6.2). It opens into the infundibulum and consequently into the hiatus semilunaris. The nasolacrimal duct is located an average of 4 mm anterior to this ostium, an important consideration in surgical enlargement of the ostium.[11]

The natural ostium of the maxillary sinus is an elliptical opening of variable size. In 15% to 40% of sinuses an accessory or secondary ostium is identified,[12] and may be found in the infundibulum or membranous fontanelle. This fontanelle is a dehiscence in the bony medial wall of the maxillary sinus, and is covered with a membrane. Accessory openings in this fontanelle are frequently associated with chronic infectious processes of the antrum.

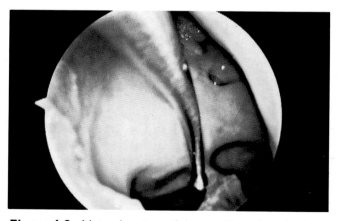

Figure 6.2. Natural ostium of the maxillary sinus (cadaver dissection).

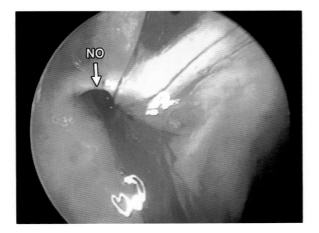

Figure 6.3. Endoscopy of the maxillary sinus. Blood-stained mucus transported toward the natural ostium. (NO = natural ostium).

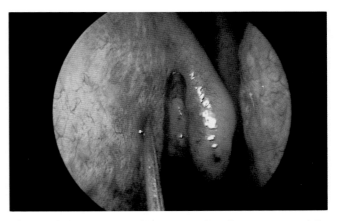

Figure 6.4. Injection of lateral nasal wall at junction of the uncinate process.

Secretions within the maxillary antrum are transported via an active mechanism from the floor of the sinus in a stellate pattern toward the natural ostium (Figure 6.3). This mucus is moved from all internal surfaces of the sinus, converging at the natural ostium in the medial wall.[13] Once the secretion passes through the ostium, it moves through a series of narrow passages before exiting into the nasal cavity. The maxillary sinus ostium normally opens into the floor of the posterior third of the infundibulum. This structure is bounded by the uncinate process medially and the lamina papyracea laterally. The infundibulum then opens into the middle meatus through the hiatus semilunaris. Secretions are next transported over the medial face of the inferior turbinate, and then posteriorly into the nasopharynx.[13]

SURGICAL APPROACHES

Hemostasis

As with all sinus techniques, it is critical to have a bloodless field for safe and effective surgery. Cotton pledgets lightly saturated with 1:1,000 epinephrine are inserted into the nares along the middle turbinate and parallel to the middle meatus. These pledgets are then left in position for 5 to 10 min. The pledgets are removed, and injections are made using

1% xylocaine with 1:100,000 epinephrine. These injections are made into several areas. First, an injection is made along the lateral wall of the nose, at the junction with the uncinate process (Figure 6.4). Injection is then made at the insertion of the middle turbinate into the lateral wall of the nose, and also into the anterior surface of the middle turbinate (Figure 6.5). These injections are made submucosally, and a blanching of the mucosa can be appreciated with the injection. Finally, an injection is made beneath the middle turbinate in the area of the exit

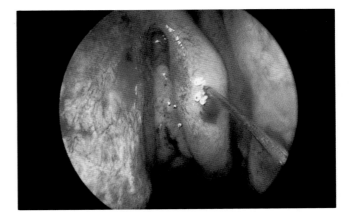

Figure 6.5. Injection of anterior surface of the middle turbinate.

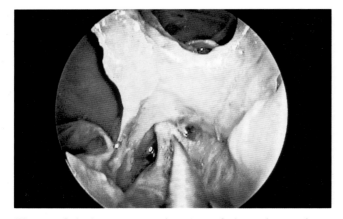

Figure 6.6. Injection at the exit of the sphenopalatine artery.

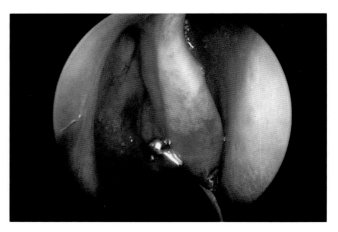

Figure 6.7. Ball probe placed posteriorly to identify the uncinate process.

of the sphenopalatine artery into the nose. This location is just posterior to the posterior wall of the maxillary sinus (Figure 6.6). We have not found it necessary to inject the sphenopalatine artery intraorally through the sphenopalatine canal, as injection in this manner has been shown to have serious potential consequences.

Uncinectomy

The key landmark in approaching the maxillary ostium through the middle meatus is the uncinate process. This structure is easily identified with a blunt ball probe or Lusk seeker (Figure 6.7), and is usually more posterior than the operating surgeon initially assumes. By using the seeker, the uncinate can be tented out and its free edge and infundibulum easily identified (Figure 6.8). Using the ball probe, the uncinate is traced superiorly to identify its insertion. Stammberger identified the various insertions of the uncinate process. It can be inserted laterally into the lateral nasal wall, vertically to the skull base, or medially toward the middle turbinate.[13] This anatomy is important in that the infundibulum, when the uncinate inserts laterally, will end in a blind pouch, referred to as the *recessus terminalis*. The frontal sinus, therefore, will usually drain directly into the middle meatus rather than

into the infundibulum, making frontal sinus disease less common with this anatomic configuration. Also, irregularities of the uncinate such as a medially bent uncinate (Figure 6.9), a pneumatized uncinate (Figure 6.10), a laterally displaced and adherent uncinate, and uncinate duplication (Figure 6.11) can be identified with the ball probe and visualized.

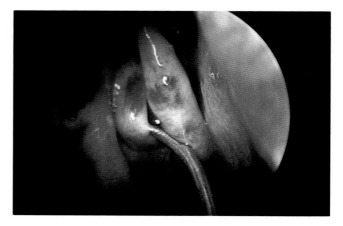

Figure 6.8. Ball probe placed posteriorly to identify the uncinate process.

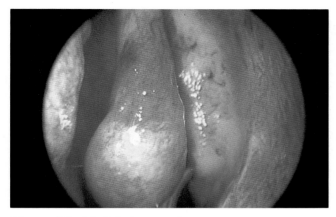

Figure 6.9. Medially bent uncinate process.

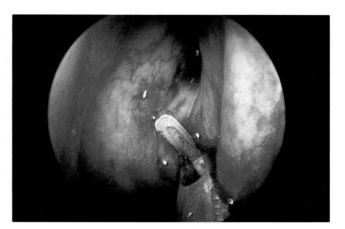

Figure 6.12. Side biting forceps used to create window in the uncinate process.

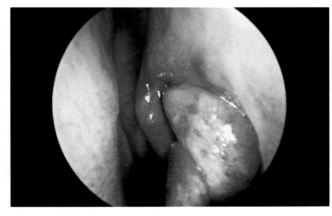

Figure 6.10. Pneumatized uncinate process.

At this point, a rough surface is needed for the microdebrider to purchase. A small window can therefore be taken out of the uncinate process with a side biting forceps, creating this rough edge (Figures 6.12, 6.13, 6.14). This step allows dissection and removal of the uncinate process both inferiorly and

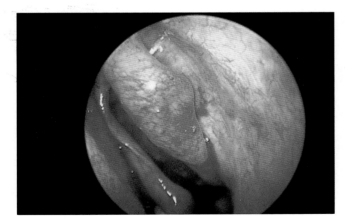

Figure 6.11. Duplication of the uncinate process.

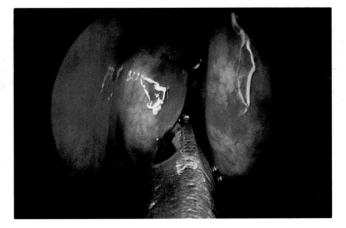

Figure 6.13. Side biting forceps used to create window in the uncinate process.

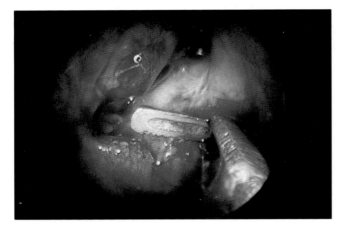

Figure 6.14. Side biting forceps used to create window in the uncinate process.

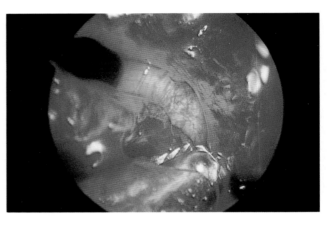

Figure 6.16. Natural ostium of the maxillary sinus.

superiorly. An alternate technique would be to make a small tear in the uncinate process from lateral to medial using the ball probe, thereby creating this rough edge for the microdebrider to capture. Using a gentle rolling motion, the uncinate process can be easily and completely removed (Figure 6.15). Adequate suction and a rough surface on which the

unit can purchase are the keys to this dissection. We prefer using the double serrated 4-mm bit. It is critical to remove the inferior portion of the uncinate process, as the natural ostium will be found in this area (Figure 6.16). Failure to remove this remnant (Figure 6.17) thoroughly is a frequent cause of persistent and recurrent maxillary sinusitis.

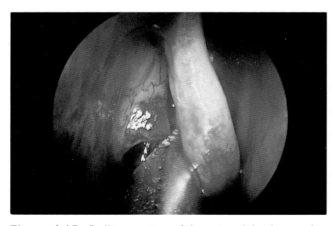

Figure 6.15. Rolling motion of the microdebrider used to remove the uncinate process.

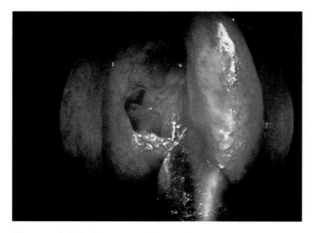

Figure 6.17. Removal of the inferior uncinate remnant.

Maxillary Antrostomy

On removal of the inferior uncinate process, the ball probe can often be inserted directly into the natural ostium and its patency assessed (Figure 6.18). It is important to remember that the natural ostium is usually in an oblique plane extending inferolaterally from its middle meatal opening (Figure 6.19). Care must therefore be taken to follow this inferolateral plane in order to avoid entry into the orbit from a more superior dissection. Once the natural ostium is identified, using the ball probe a small tear can be made inferiorly giving a rough surface for the microdebrider to purchase (Figure 6.20).

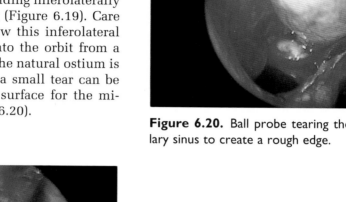

Figure 6.20. Ball probe tearing the ostium of the maxillary sinus to create a rough edge.

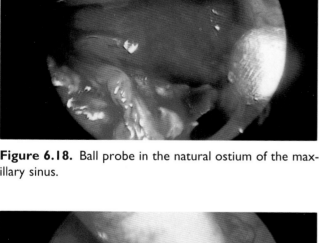

Figure 6.18. Ball probe in the natural ostium of the maxillary sinus.

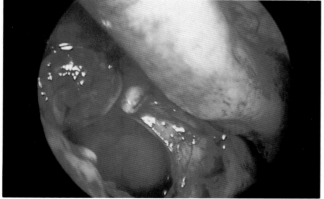

Figure 6.19. Natural ostium of the maxillary sinus lying on an oblique plane extending inferolaterally.

Enlargement of the natural ostium had traditionally been described in an anterior direction with back-biting forceps. This procedure would frequently cause disruption of the nasolacrimal duct. Using the present technique, the ostium is enlarged posteriorly (Figures 6.21 and 6.22) and inferiorly (Figures 6.23 and 6.24), thereby protecting the nasolacrimal duct anteriorly and any injury to the orbital floor superiorly. At this point, again a gentle wiping motion is used with the microdebrider to remove tissue and widen the ostium to the desired diameter. This procedure can be done using a straight bit, however newly designed instrumentation has facilitated the dissection. This new bit has a 15° curve with a small window on the convex surface (Figures 6.25 and 6.26), allowing easier and safer dissection in a posterior and inferior orientation. Using the newly designed convex surface cutting bit, one is able to dissect and enlarge the maxillary ostium "on the push" posteriorly and inferiorly. This maneuver results in very little denuded tissue (Figure 6.27) and decreases the reepithelialization needed for satisfactory healing.

It is essential to be sure that the natural ostium is incorporated with the newly enlarged ostium to prevent the phenomenon of mucous recirculation. It is equally important to connect any accessory maxillary ostium with the surgically enlarged middle meatal antrostomy to prevent a similar problem with

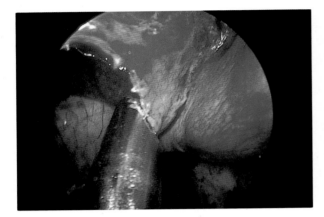

Figure 6.21. Enlargement of the maxillary ostium posteriorly.

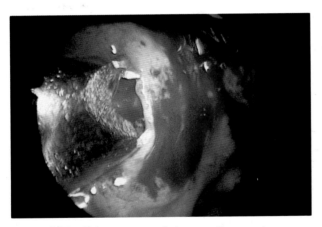

Figure 6.22. Enlargement of the maxillary ostium posteriorly.

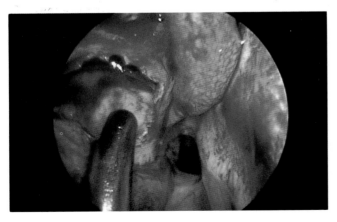

Figure 6.23. Enlargement of the maxillary ostium inferiorly.

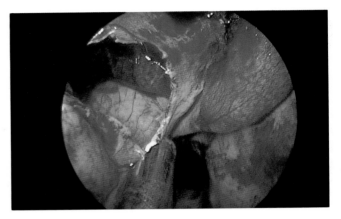

Figure 6.24. Enlargement of the maxillary ostium inferiorly.

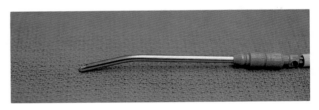

Figure 6.25. Maxillary ostium microdebrider bit with convex cutting window.

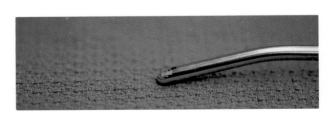

Figure 6.26. Maxillary ostium microdebrider bit with convex cutting window.

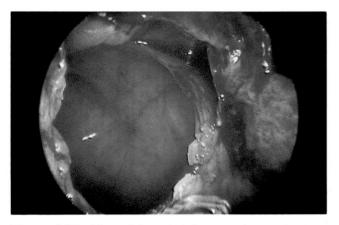

Figure 6.27. Minimal deepithelialization of normal mucosa in the ostium.

recirculation (Figure 6.28). In addition, consideration needs to be given to the clinical situation in which an inferior antrostomy exists. In these circumstances, recirculation between the inferior and middle antrostomies can occur, and can be a source of persistent disease and surgical failure. The surgeon will need to consider whether a connection

should be made between these two openings in order to prevent this phenomenon.

Maxillary sinusotomy or middle meatal antrostomy is performed easily with the microdebrider for a variety of pathologic situations. These circumstances include aeration and ventilation for inflammatory disease, both chronic and refractory acute processes (Figure 6.29). Polypoid disease of the maxillary antrum can be approached with the microdebrider as well.

Fungal Sinusitis

Allergic fungal sinusitis is one type of pathology which frequently involves the maxillary antrum. The occurrence of fungal balls and inspissated fungal secretion is commonly noted in the antrum (Figure 6.30), and can be difficult to exenterate adequately. Making a wide antrostomy (Figure 6.31) with the microdebrider gives good access to the maxillary sinus through the middle meatus, and significantly lessens the necessity of performing a Caldwell-Luc procedure for approaching this area. In addition, as bit design improves, the fungal debris will be easily removed through this antrostomy utilizing the microdebrider as the primary instrument for this procedure (Figure 6.32).

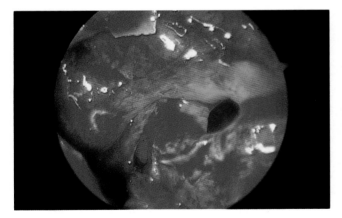

Figure 6.28. Accessory ostium of the maxillary sinus.

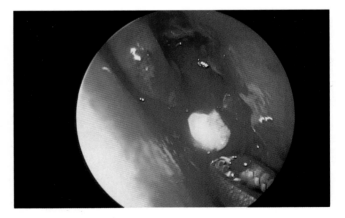

Figure 6.29. Acute maxillary sinusitis with purulent discharge.

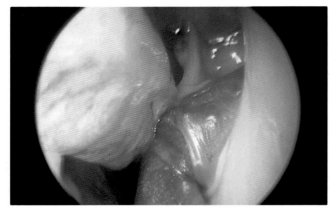

Figure 6.30. Fungal debris in the maxillary antrum.

Antral Polyps and Cysts

Polypoid disease near the antrostomy (Figure 6.33) can be removed directly with a microdebrider with minimal trauma and bleeding. The polypoid tissue is suctioned toward the ostium and removed with the action of the powered device. With modifications in bit design currently under development, large polypoid masses in the maxillary antrum will be able to be easily removed with the microdebrider (Figures 6.34, 6.35, 6.36).

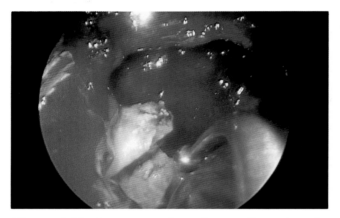

Figure 6.31. Antrostomy into the maxillary sinus for removal of fungal debris.

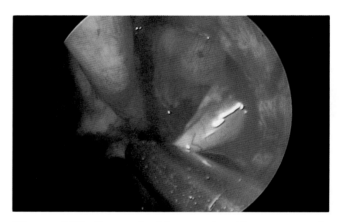

Figure 6.33. Removal of large polypoid mass near the maxillary ostium.

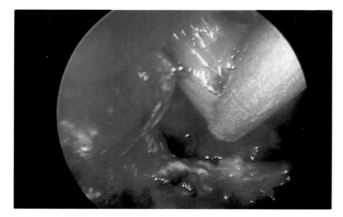

Figure 6.32. Microdebrider removing the fungal debris from the maxillary antrum.

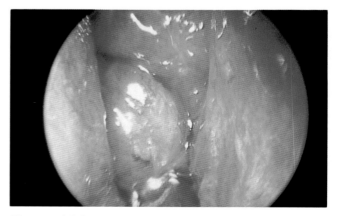

Figure 6.34. Microdebrider removing polypoid tissue from the maxillary antrum.

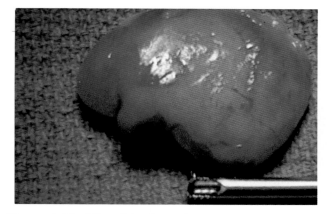

Figure 6.35. Microdebrider with polypoid tissue from the maxillary antrum.

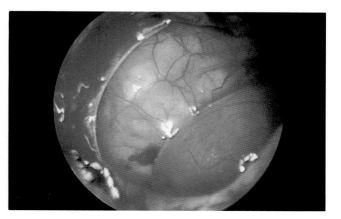

Figure 6.37. Cystic mass of the maxillary antrum.

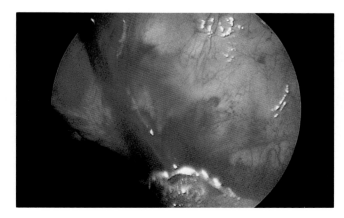

Figure 6.36. Microdebrider removing polypoid tissue from the maxillary antrum.

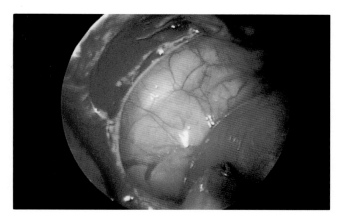

Figure 6.38. Cystic masses of the maxillary antrum approached through the antrostomy using the microdebrider.

In addition, large cystic masses of the antrum (Figure 6.37) can be easily approached through the middle meatal antrostomy. As a large opening is created into the lateral wall of the nose with the microdebrider (Figure 6.38), the surgeon gains excellent access to the antrum, and can remove cystic disease in that area with standard instrumentation or with modified microdebrider bits (Figure 6.39). Again, the necessity of a Caldwell–Luc approach is greatly reduced through use of the present technique.

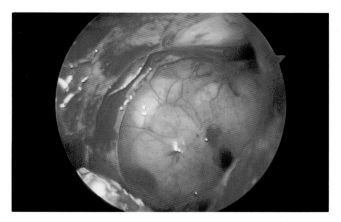

Figure 6.39. Cystic masses have been removed from the maxillary antrum.

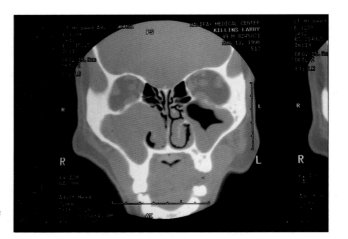

Figure 6.40. CT scan demonstrating large inverted papilloma of the maxillary sinus.

Inverted Papilloma

One indication for the microdebrider technology which remains quite controversial is the use of this device for resection of inverted (or inverting, or Schneiderian) papillomas of the ethmoid and maxillary sinuses (Figure 6.40). The microdebrider lends itself very well to the removal of soft tissue, and papillomas can be easily removed through this technique (Figures 6.41 and 6.42). With an adequate antrostomy, office endoscopy can be easily used to follow these patients postoperatively for recurrence, which can therefore be treated early if necessary. While adequate data have not been examined to support the long-term effectiveness of this procedure, reports from several surgeons have indicated that in those patients in whom it is felt that complete dissection is possible with this technique, the use of the microdebrider can save them from an open and possibly more morbid procedure.[14–15] Additional research will be necessary to further explore the utility of the microdebrider technique in these patients.

CONCLUSION OF THE MAXILLARY DISSECTION

A rolled Gelfilm splint is usually placed in the middle meatus between the middle turbinate and the lateral wall of the nose (Figure 6.43). It is important not to totally occlude the maxillary ostium with the splint. This placement can be easily accomplished by viewing the splint from below with a 30° 4-mm telescope after the splint has been inserted (Figure 6.44). Attention to detail in placing the splint minimizes discomfort to the patient in the postoperative period and probably decreases granulation tissue formation. Ostial occlusion following surgery has been attributed to inaccurate placement of this stent.[16]

Bleeding in powered dissection of the maxillary sinus rarely necessitates cauterization. The minimal bleeding and attention to securing excellent hemostasis also means that nasal packing is not necessary. The patient therefore will experience less discomfort. Powered dissection represents a safer and improved technique for maxillary sinus surgery.

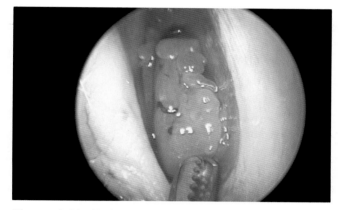

Figure 6.41. Endoscopic view of inverted papilloma.

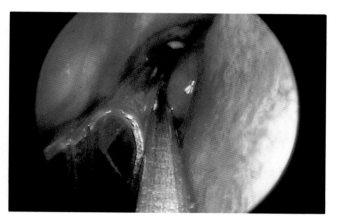

Figure 6.43. Splint inserted into the middle meatus.

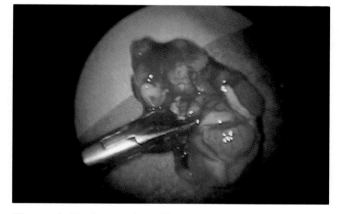

Figure 6.42. Inverted papilloma gross specimen.

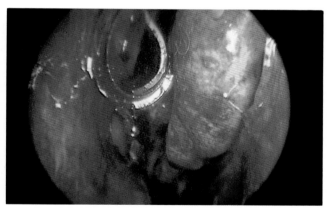

Figure 6.44. Splint shown not to occlude the maxillary ostium inferior to the splint.

REFERENCES

1. Bryan JH: Diagnosis and treatment of abscess of the antrum. *JAMA* 13:478–483, 1889.
2. Caldwell GW: Diseases of the accessory sinuses of the nose and an improved method of treatment for suppuration of the maxillary antrum. *NY J Med* 58:526–528, 1893.
3. Luc H: Une nouvelle methode operatoire pour la cure radicale et rapide de l'empyeme chronique du sinus maxillaire. *Arch Laryngol (Paris)* 10: 273–285, 1897.
4. Macbeth R: Caldwell, Luc, and their operation. *Laryngoscope* 81:1652–1657, 1971.
5. Hilding AC: Physiologic basis of nasal operations. *Calif Med J* 72:103–107, 1950.
6. Hilding AC: Experimental sinus surgery: effects of operative windows on normal sinuses. *Ann Otol* 50:379–392, 1941.
7. Messerklinger W: Uber die Drainage der men-

schlichen Nasennebenhohlen unter normalen und pathologischen Benkingungen: II. Mitteilung: Die Stirnhohle und ihr Ausfuhrungssystem. *Monatsschr Ohrenheilkd* 101:313–326, 1967.

8. Wigand ME, Steiner W: Endonasale Kieferhohlenoperation mit endoskopischer Kontrolle. *Laryngol Rhinol Otol (Stuttg)* 56:421–425, 1977.

9. Kennedy DW: Functional endoscopic sinus surgery. *Arch Otolaryngol* 111:643–649, 1985.

10. Van Alyea OE: *Nasal Sinuses: An Anatomic and Clinical Consideration,* ed 2. Baltimore, Williams & Wilkins, 1951.

11. Lang J: *Clinical Anatomy of the Nose, Nasal Cavity and Paranasal Sinuses.* New York, Thieme Medical Publishers, 1989.

12. Rice DH, Schaefer SD: *Endoscopic Paranasal Sinus Surgery.* ed 2. New York, Raven Press, 1993.

13. Stammberger H: *Functional Endoscopic Sinus Surgery: The Messerklinger Technique.* Philadelphia, Decker, 1991.

14. Waitz G, Wigand ME: Results of endoscopic sinus surgery for the treatment of inverted papillomas. *Laryngoscope* 102:917–920, 1992.

15. Kamel RH: Conservative endoscopic surgery in inverted papilloma. *Arch Otolaryngol Head Neck Surg* 118:649–653, 1992.

16. Stankiewicz J: Personal communication. Oct. 1, 1996.

7

Powered Dissection of the Sphenoid Sinus

Dewey A. Christmas, Jr., M.D.
John H. Krouse, M.D., Ph.D., F.A.C.S.

BACKGROUND

Surgery on the sphenoid sinus was a relatively late development in otolaryngology, in comparison with maxillary and frontal surgery which began in the late nineteenth century.[1] The primary reason for this history was the anatomic contiguity of the sphenoid sinus with several critical structures, including the skull base, the internal carotid artery, and the optic nerve. Experience had been gained by otolaryngologists with the recently developed Caldwell–Luc procedure,[2,3] and during the early 1900s surgeons became more comfortable with operating in the sinuses. The first approaches to the sphenoid sinus were conducted through the maxillary antrum, due in large part to the popularity of the Caldwell–Luc technique.[4]

It was only after comfort was gained with intranasal surgery in the years between 1912 and 1929 that sphenoidotomy performed through a transnasal route became accepted. Standard sphenoethmoidectomy techniques were popularized during this period, and became widely practiced over the succeeding years. With the development of nasal endoscopes, this procedure became safer and more easily performed, with a subsequent additional increase in its popularity. Wigand[5] described his approach to endoscopic sphenoid surgery, and additional modifications were added by Stammberger.[6]

ANATOMY AND PHYSIOLOGY

The sphenoid sinus is seen as an evagination of the sphenoethmoid recess at birth. It begins to develop at about age 3, pneumatizing the sphenoid bone, and by age 7 the sphenoid sinus extends posteriorly toward the sella turcica.[7] There is extensive variation in the size of the sinus with pneumatization often extending into the surrounding bony structures of the head. The sinus is divided into right and left chambers by a septum which can be quite variable in its location, resulting in large differences in the volume of each sinus.

The adult sphenoid sinus is of variable size. As it expands laterally, vessels and nerves in the lateral aspect of the sphenoid bone form indentations into the walls of the sinus. Van Alyea[8] found that in 65% of cadaver specimens the internal carotid artery formed a projection into the lateral wall of the sphenoid sinus. In addition, Dixon[9] reported that the optic nerve provided an indentation into the lateral wall of the sinus in 8% of specimens. At times these structures thin the overlying bone significantly, resulting in very little protection from trauma during surgical approaches to the sphenoid sinus. In fact, frank dehiscence of the lateral wall over these structures can be encountered during surgery.

The natural ostium of the sphenoid sinus is located at its superior aspect anteriorly, and drains

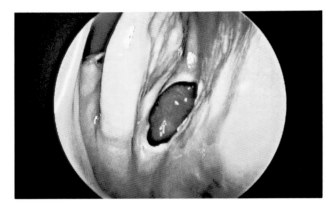

Figure 7.1. Sphenoethmoid recess showing superior turbinate and natural sphenoid ostium.

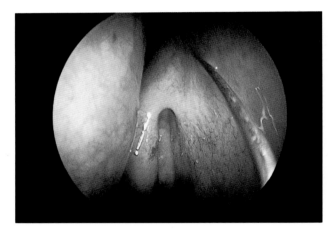

Figure 7.2. Injection of lateral nasal wall.

into the sphenoethmoid recess (Figure 7.1). The ostium is generally 2 to 3 mm in diameter, and may be round or elliptical.[8] Both Stammberger[6] and Rice and Schaefer[7] point out that the location of the sphenoid sinus and its ostium is often more inferior than the surgeon might expect. As with the other sinuses, the sphenoid sinus depends on active mucociliary transport for drainage. In this sinus, there is a spiral transportation of mucus toward the ostium which then passes into the sphenoethmoidal recess.[6] Secretion from this area then passes toward the nasopharynx, sweeping over the torus tubarius on its passage inferiorly.

SURGICAL APPROACHES

Hemostasis

It is important to secure a bloodless field for a safe approach to the sphenoid sinus. In addition to the routine injection of the lateral nasal wall (Figure 7.2) and middle turbinate, it is important to control bleeding from the anterior face of the sphenoid sinus. A cotton pledget with 1:1,000 epinephrine can be placed against the anterior face of the sinus and into the sphenoethmoidal recess and left in position for 5 to 10 min. On removal of the cotton, the anterior face of the sphenoid, posterior septum, and superior turbinate are injected submucosally

with 1% xylocaine and 1:100,000 epinephrine (Figure 7.3). Small branches of the sphenopalatine artery are located along the surface of the sphenoid anteriorly. These vessels can be troublesome, and their control with excellent hemostatic technique is of great benefit.

Hemostasis can be established as the dissection is performed through the use of topical epinephrine on cotton pledgets applied to the mucosal edges throughout the surgical procedure.

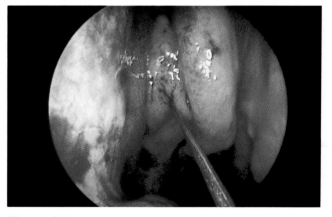

Figure 7.3. Injection of the anterior face of the sphenoid sinus.

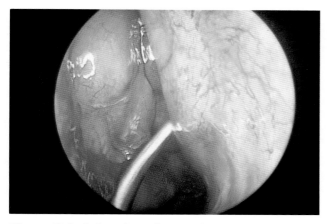

Figure 7.4. Ball probe reflecting the uncinate process.

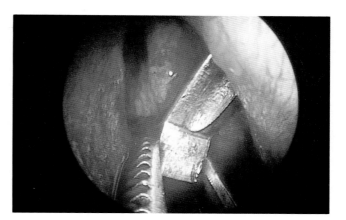

Figure 7.6. Side-biting forceps inserted behind uncinate process.

Transethmoid Sphenoidotomy

The sphenoid sinus can be approached surgically in one of two ways. In the first method, the uncinate is identified (Figures 7.4 and 7.5) and removed with the microdebrider (Figures 7.6–7.11). The ethmoid bulla (Figure 7.12) and anterior ethmoid cells are then removed from anteriorly to posteriorly (Figure 7.13). The skull base is identified and skeletonized (Figure 7.14). Dissection of the sphenoid sinus is then conducted through the posterior ethmoid cells which have been previously removed with the mi-

crodebrider. This approach is used when ethmoid surgery is indicated in the patient with both ethmoid and sphenoid disease. Once the ethmoid dissection is completed (Figure 7.15), the sphenoid sinus is approached from the most inferior and medial portion of the posterior ethmoid sinus (Figure 7.16). The posterior ethmoid cells often pneumatize extensively in a superolateral orientation, and it is in this more lateral portion of the sinus that injury to the optic nerve is most common. It is therefore prudent to establish the dissection in the inferomedial portion of the posterior ethmoid system.

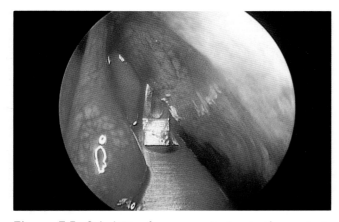

Figure 7.5. Side-biting forceps posterior to the uncinate process.

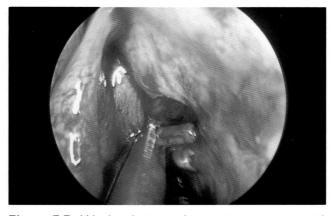

Figure 7.7. Window being made in uncinate process with side-biting forceps.

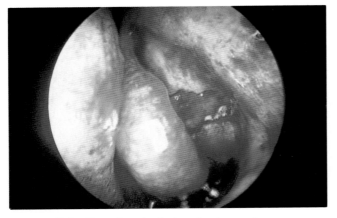

Figure 7.8. Completed window in the uncinate process, allowing grasping surface for microdebrider.

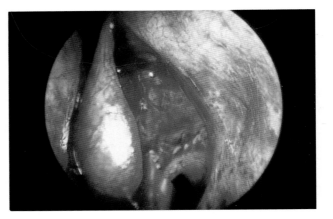

Figure 7.11. Inferior uncinate remnant being removed with the microdebrider.

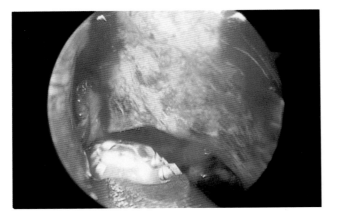

Figure 7.9. Superior portion of the uncinate process being removed with the microdebrider.

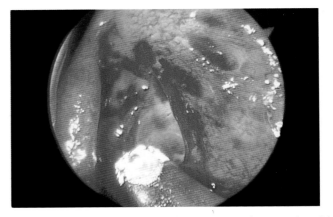

Figure 7.12. Microdebrider being inserted into ethmoid bulla.

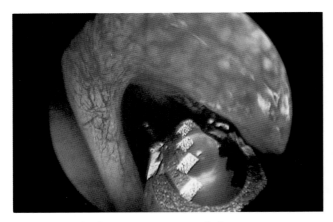

Figure 7.10. Superior portion of the uncinate process being removed with the microdebrider.

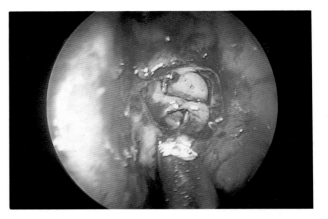

Figure 7.13. Ethmoid cells being removed anteriorly to posteriorly using the microdebrider.

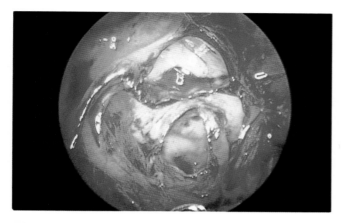

Figure 7.14. Skeletonized skull base and ethmoid roof.

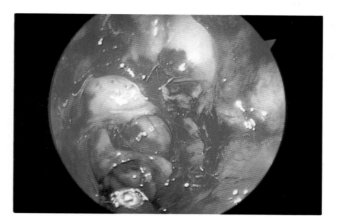

Figure 7.16. Most inferior and lateral portion of posterior ethmoid dissection.

In this region, the location of the sphenoid sinus can be easily established through gently displacing the superior turbinate from its attachment to the anterior face of the sphenoid sinus. This landmark has been described as "Parsons' ridge,"[10] from the ridge-like prominence which remains once the superior turbinate is fractured (Figure 7.17). Under endoscopic visualization, the superior turbinate, which forms the medial wall of the posterior ethmoid sinuses, can be fractured medially using a Freer elevator or the microdebrider, thus exposing this ridge. The area of the ridge provides a safe entry into the

sphenoid sinus, and is a secure and constant landmark for this procedure. If the natural ostium of the sinus can be identified at this time (Figure 7.18), it provides additional security for the surgeon that the level of the anterior face of the sphenoid sinus has been accurately identified.

The microdebrider is then used to punch into the anterior face of the sphenoid sinus in this location (Figure 7.19). It is rotated circumferentially to enlarge the surgical opening (Figure 7.20), allowing creation of a patent sphenoid ostium. Once the opening has been enlarged sufficiently, it is prudent

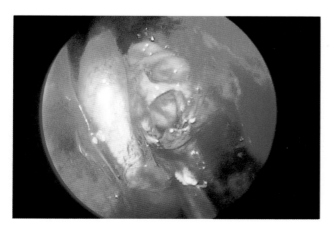

Figure 7.15. Completed ethmoid dissection.

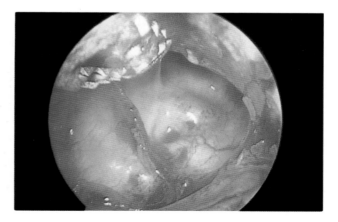

Figure 7.17. Parsons' ridge (insertion of superior turbinate to anterior sphenoid face).

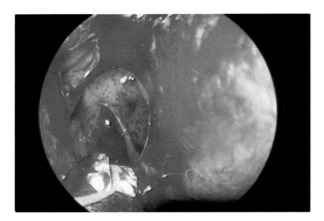

Figure 7.18. Natural ostium of the sphenoid sinus (identified in upper left portion of image).

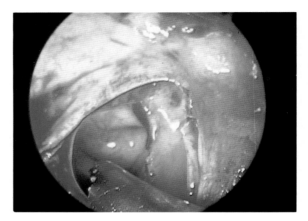

Figure 7.20. Circumferential enlargement of the sphenoid opening.

to visualize the lateral sphenoid wall with the endoscope (Figure 7.21) in order to localize the optic nerve canal and carotid artery (Figure 7.22). Often a depression can be seen between the optic canal superiorly and the carotid canal inferiorly. This depression defines the infraoptic recess (Figure 7.23).

A rough edge had been previously created through entering into the sphenoid sinus, allowing the dissecting window of the microdebrider to adequately purchase the tissue (Figure 7.24). In addition, the

current 4-mm doubly serrated bits (Figure 7.25) allow for an easier dissection of the bony face of the sinus, and can be used with a back-and-forth action (Figure 7.26) to gently file this bone, combined with a side-to-side rolling action (Figure 7.27) for tissue removal. Bits of longer length are under development to allow easier dissection in those cases with greater distances to the anterior sphenoid wall from the anterior nasal spine. These bits will allow better maneuverability of the microdebrider

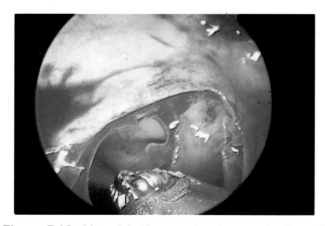

Figure 7.19. Microdebrider entering the anterior face of the sphenoid through the posterior ethmoid sinuses.

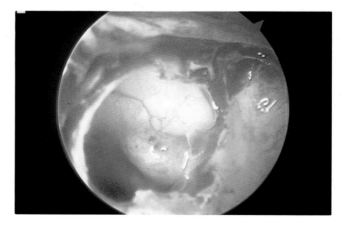

Figure 7.21. Visualization of the lateral sphenoid wall.

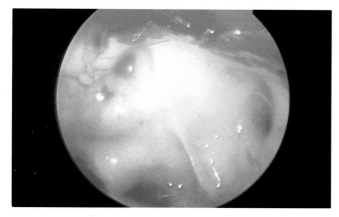

Figure 7.22. View of the optic nerve canal superiorly and the carotid artery inferiorly.

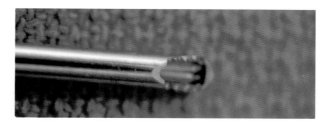

Figure 7.25. 4-mm double serrated cutting bit.

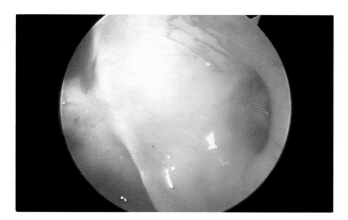

Figure 7.23. Infraoptic recess.

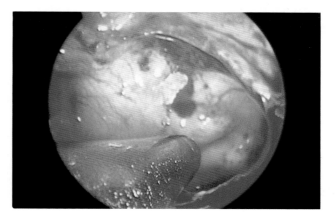

Figure 7.26. Back-and-forth motion of the microdebrider bit.

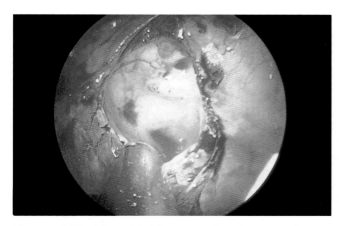

Figure 7.24. Microdebrider removing tissue at the entrance to the sphenoid sinus.

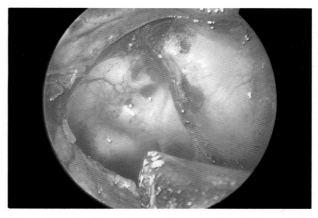

Figure 7.27. Side-to-side rolling motion of the microdebrider bit.

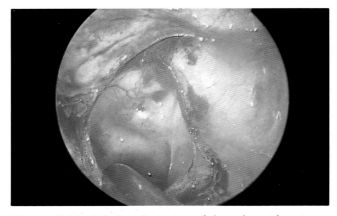

Figure 7.28. Inferior dissection of the sphenoid ostium.

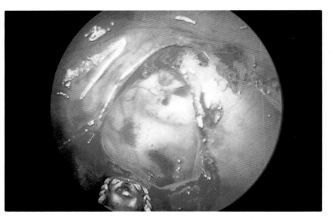

Figure 7.30. Completed dissection viewed through the posterior ethmoid opening.

handpiece without interference with the endoscope and crowding of the instruments at the entry to the nasal cavity.

It is important to remember that the dissection should always remain below the level of the natural ostium of the sphenoid. Dissection can therefore be carried out inferiorly (Figure 7.28), and lateral and medial (Figure 7.29) to the natural ostium of the sphenoid sinus. Direct visualization of this procedure is carried out at all times, allowing safe dissection with avoidance of injury to the important structures in the lateral sphenoid wall. With this close observation of the lateral sphenoid wall, the dissec-

tion can be safely completed (Figures 7.30 and 7.31). It is important to remember that if a natural ostium can be identified it should be included in the surgical window in order to prevent the phenomenon of recirculation of mucus secretion between the natural and surgical openings.

Transnasal Sphenoidotomy

An alternate approach to the sphenoid sinus can be performed through a direct transnasal route to the anterior sphenoid face. The sphenoid sinus is first

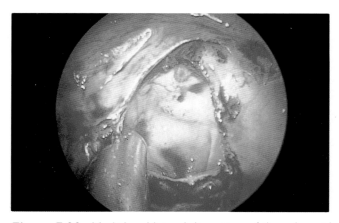

Figure 7.29. Medial and lateral dissection of the sphenoid opening.

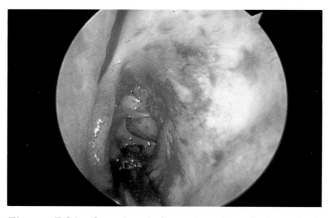

Figure 7.31. Completed dissection viewed through the middle meatus.

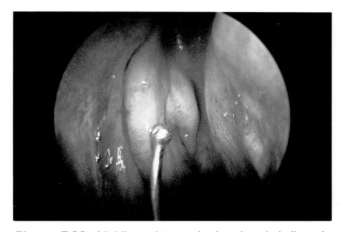

Figure 7.32. Middle turbinate displaced with ball probe showing superior turbinate.

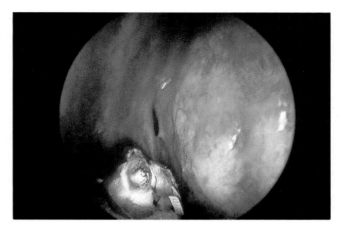

Figure 7.34. View of the right sphenoid ostium and septum medially and superior turbinate laterally.

identified through the nose by locating the superior turbinate (Figure 7.32 and 7.33). This process can be done easily through displacing the middle turbinate laterally with the shaft of the microdebrider. The natural ostium of the sphenoid sinus is usually found between the attachment of the superior turbinate laterally and the posterior nasal septum medially (Figure 7.34). The ostium is usually located in a narrow cleft formed by these bordering structures (Figure 7.35). If the natural ostium cannot be identified visually, displacement of the superior turbinate laterally can be performed, thereby fracturing it lat-

erally from its inferior insertion. The area of the insertion is Parsons' ridge, previously described in the transethmoid approach to the sphenoid sinus. Safe entry can always be made in the area of this ridge when the natural ostium is not visible. An alternate technique is to resect the inferior border of the superior turbinate with the microdebrider, thus exposing its inferior insertion (Figures 7.36–7.38).

The microdebrider is then used for dissection either through the natural ostium or through the area of the insertion of the superior turbinate. Again the microdebrider can be used to punch through into the

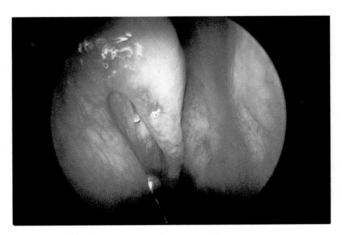

Figure 7.33. Superior turbinate with superior meatus.

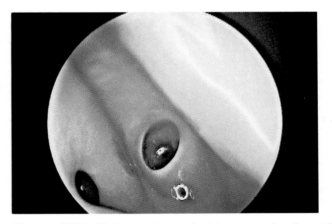

Figure 7.35. Cadaver view of right natural sphenoid ostium.

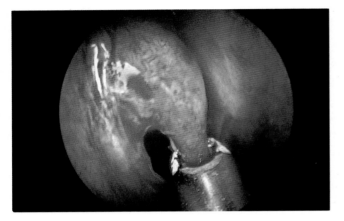

Figure 7.36. Microdebrider grasping inferior edge of right superior turbinate.

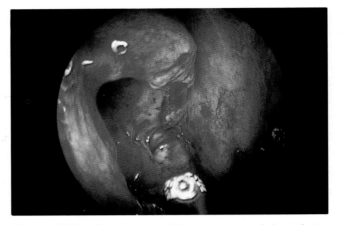

Figure 7.38. Completion of the resection of the inferior portion of the right superior turbinate, showing anterior face of sphenoid and natural sphenoid ostium.

sphenoid sinus (Figure 7.39). It is essential to examine the inside of the sinus at this point in order to establish the location of the internal carotid artery and optic nerve canal (Figures 7.40 and 7.41). As noted above, the dissection should never be carried out superiorly to the uppermost portion of the natural ostium, but rather medially (Figure 7.42), laterally (Figure 7.43), and inferiorly (Figure 7.44). Using the new doubly serrated bits makes dissection of the sphenoid sinus much safer and easier (Figures 7.45 and 7.46).

The medial portion of the dissection is limited by the nasal septum. Inferior dissection is limited by the floor of the sphenoid sinus. Lateral dissection is limited by the lateral wall of the sphenoid sinus and its impressions by the optic nerve and internal carotid artery. Lateral dissection, therefore, should be carried out with great caution and only if excellent visibility is possible. Since a significant percentage of carotid arteries are dehiscent in the lateral wall of the sphenoid sinus (Figures 7.47 and 7.48), no mass in this location should be removed surgi-

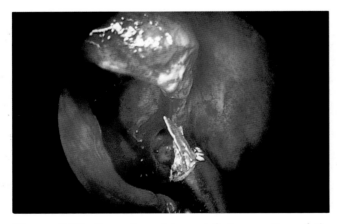

Figure 7.37. Resection of bony inferior portion of the right superior turbinate.

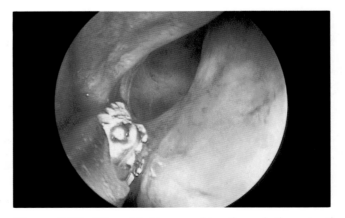

Figure 7.39. Microdebrider punching through the natural sphenoid ostium.

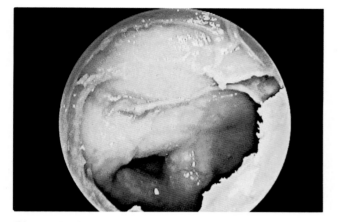

Figure 7.40. Cadaver view of right sphenoid sinus, showing optic canal superiorly and carotid artery inferiorly.

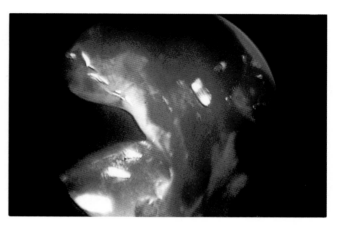

Figure 7.43. Medial dissection of the right sphenoid ostium.

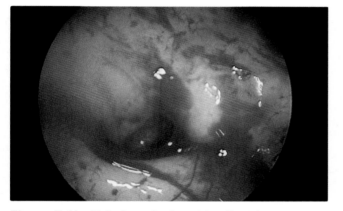

Figure 7.41. Right lateral sphenoid wall, with optic nerve canal superiorly, carotid artery inferiorly, and the infraoptic recess.

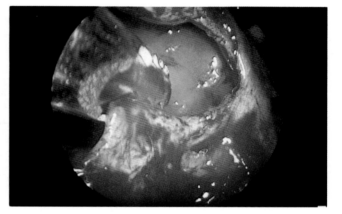

Figure 7.44. Inferior dissection of the right sphenoid ostium.

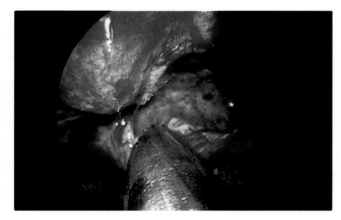

Figure 7.42. Lateral dissection of the right sphenoid ostium.

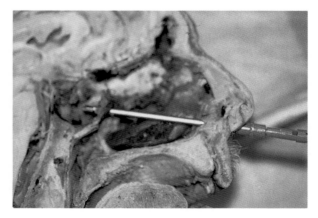

Figure 7.45. Sagittal cadaver sections demonstrating 4-mm doubly serrated blades in the sphenoid sinus.

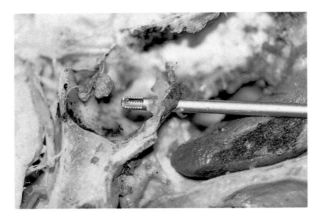

Figure 7.46. Sagittal cadaver sections demonstrating 4-mm doubly serrated blades in the sphenoid sinus.

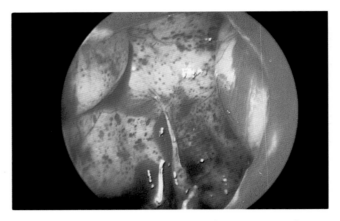

Figure 7.48. Right lateral sphenoid sinus mass, demonstrating dehiscent carotid artery.

cally with the microdebrider. Any soft tissue to be removed within the body of the sphenoid sinus (Figures 7.49 and 7.50) can be dissected with great care through the use of the microdebrider. An advantage of the powered dissection is that it does not strip out the normal mucosa from the sphenoid sinus, and therefore does not provide a large area of denuded bone which would require reepithelialization.

Conclusion of the Dissection

The surgically created ostium is generally enlarged to a diameter of at least 1 cm (Figure 7.51) to preserve long-term patency, although even larger openings can be created if necessary. A tightly rolled Gelfilm splint can be used to stent the opening and sphenoethmoidal recess area during the period of postoperative healing (Figures 7.52 and 7.53). The

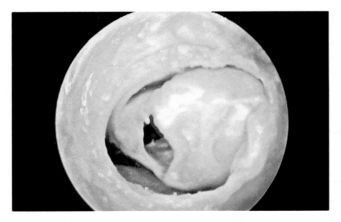

Figure 7.47. Dehiscent carotid artery filling the sphenoid sinus cavity (cadaver specimen).

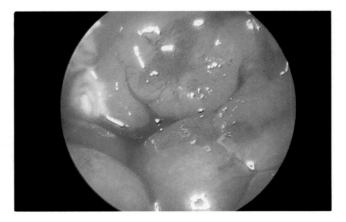

Figure 7.49. Sphenoid sinus filled with several large polypoid masses.

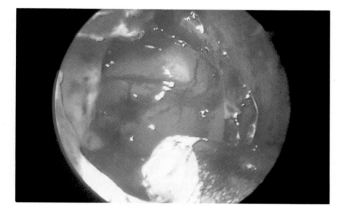

Figure 7.50. Microdebrider removing polypoid tissue from the sphenoid sinus.

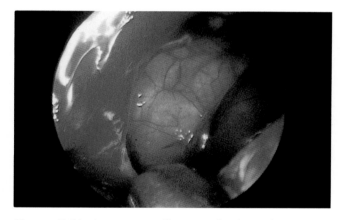

Figure 7.51. Large surgically created sphenoid ostium.

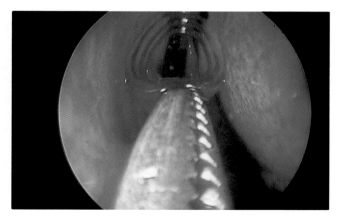

Figure 7.52. Gelfilm splint being inserted into the sphenoid ostium.

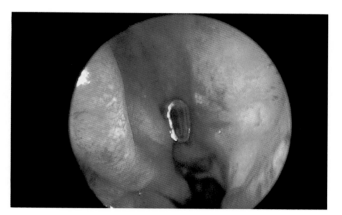

Figure 7.53. View of sphenoid splint in position in the ostium.

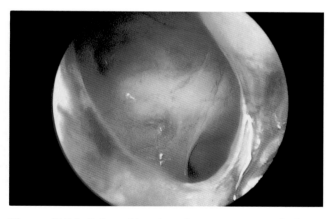

Figure 7.54. Sphenoid ostium 1 year postoperatively.

splint is generally removed in 1 to 2 weeks in the office. This procedure allows a nicely patent ostium, and heals without significant circumferential stenosis. Long-term follow-up has not demonstrated any significant stenosis of these ostia (Figure 7.54).

REFERENCES

1. Leopold D: A history of rhinology in North America. *Otolaryngol Head Neck Surg* 115:283–297, 1996.
2. Caldwell GW: Diseases of the accessory sinuses of the nose and an improved method of treat-

ment for suppuration of the maxillary antrum. *NY J Med* 58:526–528, 1893.

3. Macbeth R: Caldwell, Luc, and their operation. *Laryngoscope* 81:1652–1657, 1971.

4. Mosher HP: The anatomy of the sphenoid sinus and the method of approaching it from the antrum. *Laryngoscope* 13:177–214, 1903.

5. Wigand ME, Steiner W, Jaumann MP: Endonasal sinus surgery with endoscopial control: from radical operation to rehabilitation of the mucosa. *Endoscopy* 10:255–260, 1978.

6. Stammberger H: *Functional Endoscopic Sinus Surgery: The Messerklinger Technique.* Philadelphia, Decker, 1991.

7. Rice DH, Schaefer SD: *Endoscopic Paranasal Sinus Surgery,* ed 2. New York, Raven Press, 1993.

8. Van Alyea OE: *Nasal Sinuses: An Anatomic and Clinical Consideration,* ed 2. Baltimore, Williams & Wilkins, 1951.

9. Dixon FW: A comparative study of the sphenoid. *Ann Otol Rhinol Laryngol* 46:687–698, 1937.

10. Parsons D, Bolger W, Boyd E: The "ridge"—a safer entry to the sphenoid sinus during functional endoscopic sinus surgery in children. *Oper Tech Otolaryngol Head Neck Surg* 5:43–44, 1994.

8

Powered Instrumentation in the Management of Chronic Frontal Sinusitis

B. Manrin Rains, III

Functional endoscopic sinus surgery techniques have revolutionized and improved the surgical treatment of chronic sinusitis. In particular, endoscopic intranasal surgery of the frontal recess has significantly improved the success rate in the treatment of chronic frontal sinus disease. Endoscopic techniques have been well described by Stammberger, Kennedy, and Kuhn, as well as others.[1-6]

With the introduction of powered instrumentation in the early 1990s[7,8] and the current improvement in suction sheathed drill burs and curved blades, more precise and less traumatic frontal recess surgery is now possible. In fact, Christmas and Krouse discuss a specific approach to the frontal recess utilizing this new technology.[9] However, as taught by Stammberger[1], it is imperative to avoid mucosal injury in the frontal recess if no significant frontal sinus disease is present on initial surgery. Iatrogenic scarring and chronic frontal disease may otherwise result.

The purpose of this chapter is to discuss the endoscopic modalities of treating chronic frontal sinusitis with emphasis on powered instrumentation techniques and their benefits.

HISTORY

Intranasal and external approaches to the frontal sinus have been described since the turn of the century.[11-14] Several problems with external approaches include failure to eliminate frontal recess obstruction and destruction of the lateral bony frontal recess structures. This destruction may lead to orbital soft tissue collapse into the ethmoidectomy site resulting in frontal recess obstruction.

Osteoplastic frontal sinus obliteration with fat[15] has traditionally been the gold standard for the surgical treatment of frontal sinus disease, especially in cases of surgical failure. This procedure has significant morbidity however, and when residual or recurrent inflammatory disease occurs, evaluation is difficult, even with computed tomography (CT) follow-up.

Intranasal approaches have historically been associated with a high failure rate. Now with a better understanding of the anatomy, more delicate endoscopic techniques, and specialized instruments such as powered dissectors with curved blades and sheathed drills, the future for treating chronic frontal sinusitis has improved.

The modified transnasal endoscopic Lothrop procedure presented by Gross et al.[16-17] is a direct outgrowth of advanced drill technology and endoscopic techniques. It offers a significant alternative to osteoplastic frontal sinus obliteration with fat.

ANATOMY

Killian first used the term "frontal recess" in 1898.[10] Van Alyea's[18,19] extensive writings of 1939 through 1946 give a detailed description of a number of cells

Table 8.1. Chronic Frontal Sinusitis: The Endoscopic Frontal Recess Approach

Frontal recess cells
1. Agger nasi cell
2. Supraorbital ethmoid cells
3. Frontal cells
   a. Type I
   b. Type II
   c. Type III
   d. Type IV
4. Frontal bulla cells
5. Suprabullar cells
6. Interfrontal sinus septal cell

that potentially could obstruct the frontal sinus. These various frontal recess cells are listed in Table 8.1. Their incomplete removal at surgery and persistent chronic inflammation are causes of chronic frontal sinus obstruction and sinusitis.[2]

It is important for each endoscopic sinus surgeon to understand conceptually that there is not a "nasofrontal-duct" or tubular structure, but rather a *frontal recess* which is the area of the juncture of the frontal sinus and the anterior ethmoids. As described by Kuhn, the frontal recess is a potential, inverted, funnel-shaped space. It has a narrow upper portion at the internal frontal ostium and a lower bell-shaped end in continuity with the anterior ethmoid sinus wall (Figures 8.1 and 8.2). This funnel wall is made up superiorly by the skull base, ending near the anterior ethmoid artery. The frontal recess extends from the anterior buttress of the internal frontal ostium inferiorly to the level of the attachment of the middle turbinate. Laterally, it is bounded by the orbital plate of the frontal bone and medial orbital wall. The frontal recess is bounded medially by the vertical attachment of the middle turbinate to the skull base. This space is pneumatized by multiple anterior ethmoid cells with a widely variable pattern.[2] Every surgeon must be familiar with these anatomic variations. Correlation with CT scans and sagittal reconstruction on difficult cases is helpful.

The insertion of the uncinate process superiorly is also quite variable, and can involve one of three locations. The uncinate process can insert laterally into the lateral nasal wall, vertically to the skull

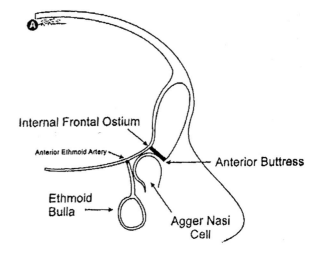

Figure 8.1. The internal frontal ostium is in a plane perpendicular to the skull base, which intersects the anterior buttress. The agger nasi cell can obstruct at the skull base or the bulla lamella. (From Kuhn FA: Chronic frontal sinusitis: The endoscopic frontal recess approach. *Oper Tech Otolaryngol Head Neck Surg* 7:221–229, 1996. Reprinted with permission.)

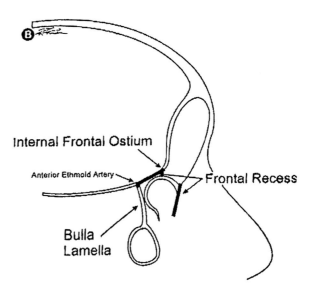

Figure 8.2. The frontal recess depicted by shaded lines is pneumatized by a large agger nasi cell. Its upper limb parallels the skull base, ending at the anterior ethmoid artery. (From Kuhn FA: Chronic frontal sinusitis: The endoscopic frontal recess approach. *Oper Tech Otolaryngol Head Neck Surg* 7:221–229, 1996. Reprinted with permission.)

base, or medially toward the middle turbinate. The location of this insertion determines the drainage pattern of the frontal sinus. If the insertion is medial or vertical to the skull base, edema or inflammation of the uncinate process is more likely to obstruct the frontal recess. It is essential therefore to remove the entire superior portion of the uncinate process to facilitate maximal drainage and ventilation of this area.

OPERATIVE TECHNIQUES

Primary Procedure

As mentioned earlier, the surgeon should not operate in the frontal recess unless significant mucosal disease is present. Postoperative scarring can result. Correlation with CT scans is always recommended in clarifying and delineating this complex anatomy. Attention must be given to identifying the opening of any midfrontal sinus cells, supraorbital cells, or interfrontal sinus septal cells. Multiple openings into the frontal recess can be present (Figures 8.3 and 8.4). The dome of the agger nasi cell must not be mistaken for the frontal sinus drainage pathway.

It is imperative to preserve the frontal recess mucous membrane. This preservation is a great advantage of powered instrumentation with curved cutting blades. Also, through-cut instrumentation and upcutting frontal recess forceps can be useful as

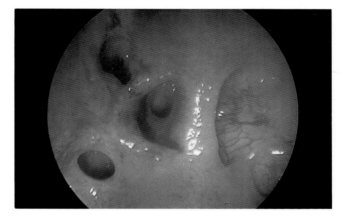

Figure 8.4. Left frontal recess in a surgical patient showing numerous openings.

adjuvant instrumentation. The Kuhn–Bolger frontal recess seeker, curettes, and forceps help remove bony lamella and spicules high in the internal frontal ostium.

In a previously unoperated patient, retrograde uncinectomy and anterior ethmoidectomy are performed as described by Christmas and Krouse.[8,20] This procedure is done using a 3.5 or 4.0-mm aggressive cutting or serrated blade. As noted earlier, it is critical to remove the entire superior portion of the uncinate process (Figures 8.5 and 8.6) to allow adequate exposure to the anterior portion of the frontal recess (Figures 8.7 and 8.8). Careful, meticulous dis-

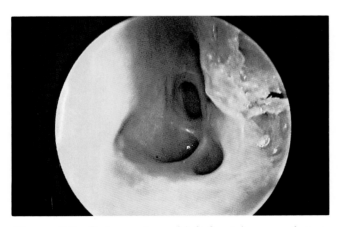

Figure 8.3. Cadaver view of left frontal recess demonstrating numerous openings superiorly.

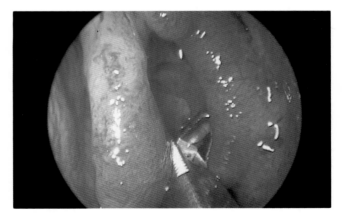

Figure 8.5. Creating window in uncinate process using side-biting forceps.

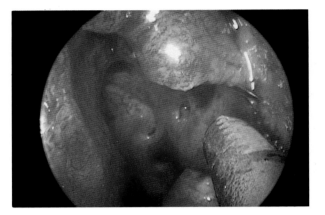

Figure 8.6. Removing superior portion of the uncinate process with the microdebrider.

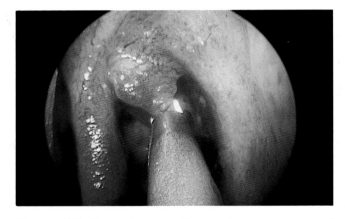

Figure 8.7. Removing superior uncinate process and opening anterior frontal recess.

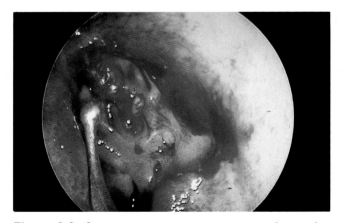

Figure 8.8. Superior uncinate process removed, revealing anterior frontal recess.

section is important in this area to avoid injury to normal mucosa and secondary stenosis.

Next, working posterior to anterior, the skull base will begin sloping sharply as the anterior ethmoid artery is approached. This is the posterior entrance to the frontal recess. A curved suction or ostia seeker can help confirm the location (Figure 8.9).

Using a curved shaver blade, the newly developed 4-mm obliquely curved shaver blades (Figures 8.10 and 8.11), or a curved curette, surgery continues anteriorly. In performing the dissection, prominent agger nasi cells are often encountered. These cells bulge from the lateral nasal wall near the insertion of the middle turbinate (Figure 8.12). The agger nasi can be entered under direct visualization through its medial and inferior walls (Figures 8.13 and 8.14),

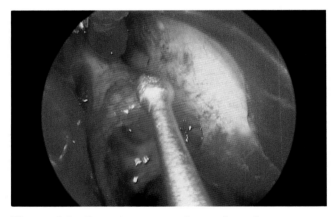

Figure 8.9. Curved ostium seeker in frontal recess.

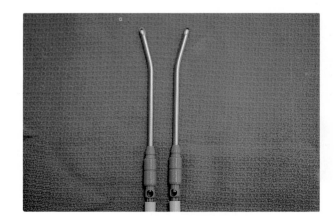

Figure 8.10. Curved, obliquely cutting frontal sinus bits.

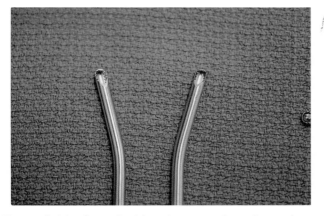

Figure 8.11. Curved, obliquely cutting frontal sinus bits.

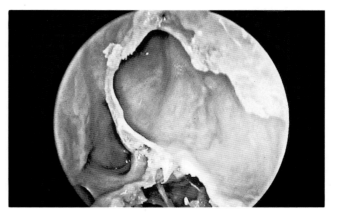

Figure 8.14. Cadaver view of large, opened left agger nasi cell.

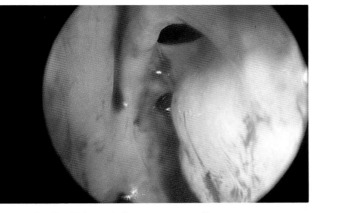

Figure 8.12. Bulging left agger nasi cell.

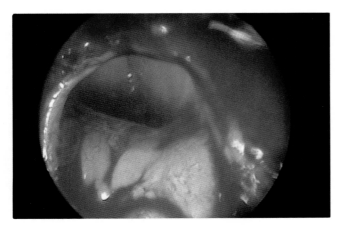

Figure 8.13. Left agger nasi cell opened with the microdebrider.

carrying the dissection anteriorly and laterally using the powered microdebrider. The inner portion of the agger nasi cell can be examined through this area, and widely opened to establish ventilation and drainage. Care must be taken to avoid working medially toward the lateral lamella of the cribriform plate or posteriorly toward the base of the skull, since these areas are most easily injured. Violation of this area will lead to intracranial penetration with its potentially serious consequences.

The frontal recess is then carefully inspected. Any polypoid masses, adhesions, mucopurulent material, or granulation tissue is noted (Figures 8.15 and 8.16). Supraorbital or other frontal cells must be opened. Using the 30° scope and the microdebrider, these various abnormalities can now be addressed, and the procedure completed (Figures 8.17 and 8.18). In patients with extensive polyposis, osteitic bone, denuded mucosa, or an extremely narrow frontal recess, a regular sized Rains frontal sinus stent can be inserted.

Postoperative follow-up with necessary debridement is performed on days 1 and 7, and on either day 14 or 21. Since using powered instrumentation, cleaning on days 14 or 21 is usually not necessary, due to faster healing felt secondary to decreased mucosal damage with the shaver (Figures 8.19 and 8.20).

Rains Frontal Sinus Stent

The Rains frontal sinus stent is a self-retaining, flexible stent of medical grade silicone rubber designed

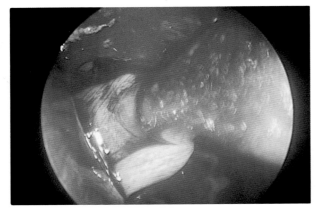

Figure 8.15. Microdebrider removing polypoid tissue from frontal recess.

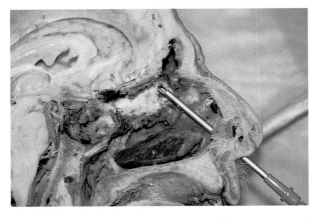

Figure 8.18. Sagittal view of completed frontal recess dissection with microdebrider bit in frontal recess (cadaver dissection).

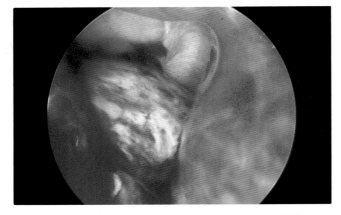

Figure 8.16. Left frontal sinus cavity visualized following removal of polypoid tissue.

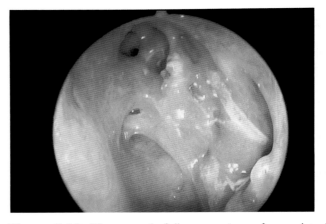

Figure 8.19. Three-week follow-up view of completed dissection of the frontal recess.

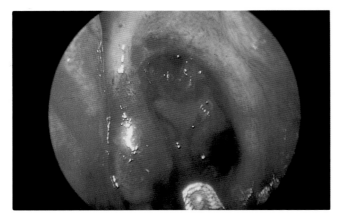

Figure 8.17. Completed dissection of the frontal recess.

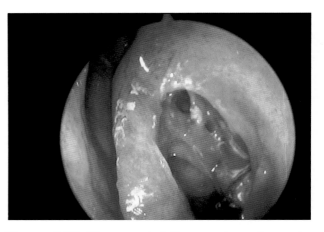

Figure 8.20. Three-week follow-up view of completed dissection of the frontal recess.

for endoscopic insertion into the frontal drainage pathway when stenting is necessary (Figure 8.21). Recommended indications for stenting include cases with extensive polypoid mucosa, osteitic bone, denuded mucosa, and a narrow frontal drainage pathway. The regular sized (4-mm) stent is easily inserted over an upcurved 16-gauge frontal sinus suction (Figures 8.22, 8.23, 8.24). It is removed in the office, when the ethmoidectomy site is healed, by grasping with small forceps. The stent is usually left in place 2–4 weeks until the ethmoid mucosa has healed. In a small number of cases with herniation of orbital contents obstructing the frontal recess (following trauma or external ethmoidectomy), the stent has remained up to 18 months thus far without problems.

The larger stent (6-mm) may be used as a frontal trephine irrigation port. It also may serve as a visualization port through the use of a pediatric 2.7-mm 70° telescope. The trephine should be 6–7 mm in diameter. It is easily made with a sheathed drill bur.

Surgical Failures and Revision Surgery

Evaluation in these cases must include a complete history and evaluation for unusual underlying medical condition such as immunoglobulin deficiencies, extensive allergies, cystic fibrosis, and ciliary dysmotility. Endoscopically guided cultures can be use-

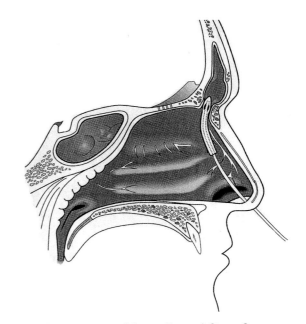

Figure 8.22. Insertion of Rains Frontal Sinus Stent over 16 gauge (#5 Fr) up-curved suction. Notice collapse of bulb section through narrowest portion of the frontal drainage pathway.

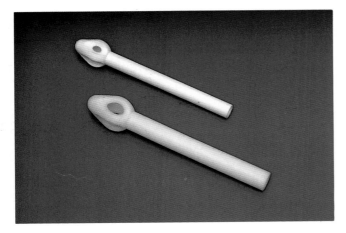

Figure 8.21. Rains Frontal Sinus Stents, 4mm and 6 mm lengths. Self-retaining, flexible, medical grade silicone rubber stents (Smith + Nephew ENT, Inc., Memphis, TN).

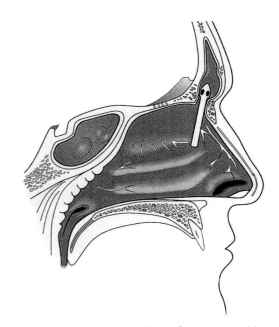

Figure 8.23. Rains Frontal Sinus Stent in position with bulb re-expanded in frontal sinus making stent self-retaining. Stent may be removed in office by grasping proximal end with a forceps.

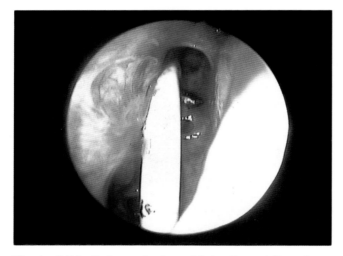

Figure 8.24. Endoscopic view of Rains Frontal Sinus Stent in position, right side.

ful in identifying antibiotic-resistant bacteria. If secretions are extremely tenacious and sticky, fungal cultures should also be obtained. If polyps are present, it is important to know their eosinophil content. If the patient has nonallergic eosinophilic rhinitis, then appropriate steroid therapy may resolve the ostial obstruction.

Coronal (3-mm cuts) and axial (3 to 5-mm cuts) CT scans are essential prior to any revision surgery. The height of the roof of the ethmoid and lateral lamella of the cribriform must be defined. It is important to note supraorbital or midfrontal sinus cells; their ostia can be opened to establish ventilation and drainage. In addition, 1-mm axial images are excellent for sagittal reconstructions which can be helpful on patients with multiple surgeries and absent anatomic landmarks. Computer-guided surgical systems can also be of assistance in these difficult cases.

Combined Endoscopic Intranasal and External Sinusotomy

In patients with recurrent disease, particularly those who have undergone previous external ethmoidectomy, the frontal recess and drainage pathway can often not be found endoscopically. In these patients, I first perform a frontal sinus trephination below the

eyebrow medially. The sheathed shaver burr makes this procedure easier because there is less chance of soft tissue catching in the drill burr. A trephination of 6–8 mm in diameter is recommended.

Next, the frontal sinus is inspected endoscopically and with irrigation or a curved probe, the frontal drainage pathway is identified using an intranasal endoscope. The frontal recess can now be opened intranasally, and if necessary, a 4-mm Rains frontal sinus stent inserted. It is important to open any frontal cells and to perform revision ethmoid surgery if disease is present.

I use a large (6-mm) Rains frontal sinus stent through the trephine as an irrigation port and for visualization with a 2.7-mm endoscope (Figure 8.1).

Modified Transnasal Endoscopic Lothrop Procedure

Draf,[22] May,[23] Wigand,[24] Close et al.,[25] and Gross et al.[16,17] have described the use of a drill transnasally to enhance frontal sinus drainage. In the modified transnasal endoscopic Lothrop procedure or frontal drill-out described by Gross et al,[16,17] a single common opening that includes both natural frontal sinus ostia is created. This maneuver should theoretically decrease the potential for mucous recirculation. Advanced powered drill technology with protective sheathing and suction, performed under endoscopic guidance, has enabled the development of this improved procedure. The beveled sheath protects the posterior table and its mucosa, helping avoid both circumferential mucosal injury and base of skull violation.

Advantages over osteoplastic frontal sinus obliteration include decreased morbidity, improved cosmesis, and cost reduction. It must be remembered that this procedure is a very technical and advanced technique to be accomplished first in the cadaver lab. It is not for the occasional endoscopic sinus surgeon, and requires extensive training and experience.

SUMMARY

Endoscopic frontal sinusotomy is rapidly becoming the gold standard for treatment of chronic frontal sinusitis. Recent technical advances of powered instrumentation improve surgical techniques in the frontal recess—first, by decreasing mucosal injury, and secondly, by facilitating new and innovative surgical procedures.

We are entering a new and more successful era in the treatment of chronic frontal sinusitis. Technology has given us new tools, but an understanding of and respect for the variable and complex anatomy of the frontal recess is vital.

REFERENCES

1. Stammberger H: *Functional Endoscopic Sinus Surgery.* Philadelphia, PA, Decker, 1991.

2. Kuhn, FA: Chronic frontal sinusitis: the endoscopic frontal recess approach. *Oper Tech Otolaryngol Head Neck Surg* 7:222–229, 1996.

3. Wigand M, Hoseman W: Endoscopic surgery for frontal sinusitis and its complications. *Am J Rhinol* 5:85–89, 1991.

4. Draf W: Endonasal micro-endoscopic frontal sinus surgery: the fulda concept. *Oper Tech Otolaryngol Head Neck Surg* 2:234–240, 1991.

5. May M: Frontal sinus surgery: endonasal endoscopic ostioplasty rather than external osteoplasty. *Oper Tech Otolaryngol Head Neck Surg* 2:247–256, 1991.

6. Kennedy DW, Zinreich SJ, Rosenbaum AE, et al: Functional endoscopic sinus surgery: theory and diagnostic evaluation. *Arch Otolaryngol* 111:576–582, 1985.

7. Setliff RC, Parsons DS: The "Hummer": new instrumentation for functional endoscopic sinus surgery. *Am J Rhinol* 8:275–278, 1994.

8. Christmas DA, Krouse JH: Powered instrumentation in functional endoscopic sinus surgery I: surgical technique. *Ear Nose Throat J* 75:33–38, 1996.

9. Christmas DA, Krouse JH: Powered instrumentation in dissection of the frontal recess. *Ear Nose Throat J* 75:425–428, 1996.

10. Killian G: Die Killan'sche Radicaloperation Chronischer Sternhohleneiterungen: II. Weiteres Kasuistisched Material und Zusammenfasung. *Arch Laryngol Rhin* 15:13–59, 1903.

11. Ingals EF: Intranasal drainage of the frontal sinus. *Ann Otol Rhinol Laryngol* 26:656–668, 1917.

12. Anderson CM: External operation on the frontal sinus: causes of failure. *Arch Otolaryngol* 15:739–745, 1932.

13. Lothrop HA: Frontal sinus suppuration with results of new operative procedure. *JAMA* 65:153–160, 1915.

14. Lynch RC: The technique of a radical frontal sinus operation, which has given me the best results. *Laryngoscope* 31:1–5, 1921.

15. Hardy JM, Montgomery WW: Osteoplastic frontal sinusotomy: analysis of 250 operations. *Ann Otolaryngol* 85:523–532, 1976.

16. Gross WE, Gross CW, Becker DG, et al: Modified transnasal endoscopic Lothrop procedure as an alternative to frontal sinus obliteration. *Otolaryngol Head Neck Surg* 113:427–434, 1995.

17. Gross CW, Gross WE, Becker DG: Modified transnasal endoscopic Lothrop procedure: frontal drill out. *Oper Tech Otolaryngol Head Neck Surg* 6:193–200, 1995.

18. Van Alyea OE: Ethmoid labyrinth: anatomic study with consideration of the clinical significance of its structural characteristics. *Arch Otolaryngol* 29:881–901, 1939.

19. Van Alyea OE: Frontal cells. *Arch Otolaryngol* 34:11–23, 1941.

20. Christmas DA, Krouse JH: Powered dissection of the ethmoid sinuses. In Krouse JH, Christmas DA: *Powered Endoscopic Sinus Surgery.* Baltimore, Williams & Wilkins, 1997.

21. Van Alyea OE: Frontal sinus drainage. *Ann Otol Rhinol Laryngol* 55:267–277, 1946.

22. Draf W: Endonasal micro-endoscopic frontal sinus surgery: the Fulda concept. *Oper Tech Otolaryngol Head Neck Surg* 2:234–240, 1991.

23. May M: Frontal sinus surgery: endonasal endoscopic ostioplasty rather than external osteoplasty. *Oper Tech Otolaryngol Head Neck Surg* 2:247–256, 1991.

24. Wigand M, Hoseman W: Endoscopic surgery for frontal sinusitis and its complications. *Am J Rhinol* 5:85–89, 1991.

25. Close LD, Lee NK, Leach JL, et al: Endoscopic resection of the intranasal frontal sinus floor. *Ann Otol Rhinol Laryngol* 103:952–958, 1994.

9

Powered Endoscopic Sinus Surgery in the Pediatric Population

James Stankiewicz, M.D.

Just as powered instrumentation is being used increasingly in adult endoscopic sinus surgery, it has also proven beneficial in pediatric endoscopic sinus surgery.[1] Powered instrumentation provides the surgeon with real-time cutting and suctioning with mucosal preservation. Since mucosal preservation is so important to appropriate, scar-free healing, it is especially important that powered instrumentation be used in the pediatric population, in which postoperative debridement can be a problem.[2] Studies have shown that the microdebrider can reduce postoperative healing time and synechia formation.[3] It is important to realize that there are anatomic differences between the adult and the child which require special instrumentation and techniques. Additionally, other considerations such as adenoid and turbinate hypertrophy, along with the location of sinus disease, may all play a role in stepwise, individualized surgery.[4] Additionally, certain other factors support a conservative approach. These factors include treatable medical problems such as gastroesophageal reflux, possible maxillary and ethmoid facial growth problems, and the fact that sinusitis, like otitis media, can be a self-limiting infection, decreasing as the child grows older.[5–7] This chapter will outline the approach to sinus surgery, discussing instrumentation, technique, and postoperative considerations. In addition, powered instrumentation has other uses in the pediatric population, such as in choanal atresia, adenoidectomy, turbinectomy, and tumor surgery. Some discussion relevant to these surgeries will also be presented.

PREOPERATIVE CONSIDERATIONS

The first goal is to decide which child is a candidate for endoscopic sinus surgery. All treatable conditions causing sinusitis need to be evaluated, diagnosed, and treated. Allergies (foods or inhalants) need to be evaluated and identified. If prolonged allergy treatment is necessary in the surgical patient who has had difficult-to-treat sinusitis and/or asthma, surgery is performed and allergy treatment is ongoing. Sinusitis and asthma are often associated disorders. Intensive medical therapy has been shown to improve sinusitus to the extent that the asthma subsides.[8] Chronic sinusitis itself (defined as the presence of symptoms for over 3 months) requires at least 6 weeks of antibiotic therapy, with consideration of a topical steroid spray or an oral steroid. Patients who fail this intensive therapy meet the relative criteria for sinus surgery. No studies are available on the role of prophylactic antibiotics in recurrent acute or chronic sinusitis. However, one study in patients with sinusitis and asthma showed some benefit.[9] Resistant bacteria due to the overuse of antibiotics, however, may temper the use of prophylaxis. Reflux esophagitis has been shown to cause sinusitis.[10] Making this diagnosis prior to potential primary or revision sinus surgeries can avoid the need for surgery. Table 9.1 shows the absolute and relative indications for endoscopic sinus surgery in children. Modifying factors such as severe allergy, immunodeficiency, mucociliary disorders, cystic fibrosis, asthma, anatomic obstruc-

Table 9.1. Absolute and Relative Indications for Sinus Surgery

Absolute Indications
  Complete nasal obstruction secondary to nasal polyps/sinusitis
  Acute sinusitis with brain abscess, meningitis, subperiosteal/
  orbital abscess, cavernous thrombosis
  Fungal sinusitis
  Sinus mucocele/pyocele
  Nasal/sinus tumor
  Cerebrospinal fluid rhinorrhea
  Meningoencephalocele
Relative Indications
  Persistent acute (uncomplicated), subacute, chronic, or
  recurrent acute sinusitis failing optimal medical therapy

Table 9.2. An Individualized, Graduated Approach to Pediatric Sinus Surgery for Chronic Sinusitis

Stage I*	Adenoidectomy
	Endoscopic sinus/nasal exam under anesthesia
	Bilateral maxillary sinus irrigation and culture
Stage II*	Limited endoscopic sinus surgery
	Anterior ethmoidectomy
	Possible maxillary antrostomy
Stage III*	Extensive endoscopic sinus surgery
	Total ethmoidectomy
	Possible maxillary antrostomy
	Frontal recess/sphenoidotomy if necessary

*Adjunctive procedures such as septoplasty or turbinate surgery can be performed, in addition, if necessary.

tions, previous sinus surgery, and previous adenoidectomy may increase the need to proceed with surgery, depending on the degree of difficulty the patient is having. Once the decision to perform surgery has been made, a surgical plan must be developed. Nasal endoscopy and computed tomography (CT) scanning can uncover anatomic variations, septal deflections, hypertrophic adenoids and turbinates, and the extent of sinus disease. On occasion, the scan can delineate a pattern of normal sinuses and nasal obstruction due to hypertrophic middle and inferior turbinates, the *halo scan,* which deserves different consideration. Also of note is that in younger children the maxillary sinus is most often involved, followed by the anterior ethmoid. Frontal and sphenoid sinusitis is uncommon.[11] As the child grows older, the ostiomeatal complex (OMC)/anterior ethmoid/maxillary sinus becomes more involved; uncommonly, sphenoid/frontal sinusitis is present. The teenage disease pattern more often follows that of the adult. Taking all of these considerations together with the need for conservation, an individualized, graduated approach for nasal and sinus surgery can be formulated (Table 9.2). Acute, complicated sinusitis is difficult to approach endoscopically because of the degree of inflammation and resultant bleeding. Powered instrumentation using the microdebrider supplies real-time suction, which can make the endoscopic approach safer. However, an external approach should always be ready as a backup procedure if appropriate drainage is not achieved.

INSTRUMENTATION

Both regular-size (4-mm) and small pediatric (2 to 2.5-mm) endoscopes are necessary to perform endoscopic nasal and sinus surgery in children. The 2.5-mm scopes are very delicate and need to be handled carefully. Pediatric endoscopic sinus surgery forceps and suctions are equally important. Small through-cutting punch forceps are also necessary. Elongated otologic instruments are extremely helpful in the small child. Pediatric backward-biting forceps are helpful and should be obtained. Most brands of microdebriders come with small tips (2.5–3.5 mm), which are necessary in the small child. Adult instrumentation can be used in the teenager in most cases. Some method of measuring distances, using either a ruler or a probe, is necessary to avoid complications. Curved small probes and suctions help to identify various areas of anatomy and can be used for gentle dissection.

PEDIATRIC SINUS SURGERY AND POWERED INSTRUMENTATION— TECHNIQUES

Adenoidectomy

Adenoidectomy should be considered if the nose is obstructed by hypertrophic adenoids or purulent adenoiditis. Adenoids can be removed in the traditional way or endoscopically via cautery or the powered microdebrider.[12] In all cases, hemostasis is important. Endoscopic removal can be performed with the endoscope and microdebrider on one side of the nose or the endoscope viewing the nasopharynx on one side and the cautery or microdebrider on the other side performing the surgery. Hemostasis is controlled with endoscopic cautery. This technique is especially helpful in the case of adenoid hypertrophy in a bifid uvula with submucous cleft palate where precise adenoid removal is necessary or in a patient with human immunodeficiency virus in whom blood loss needs to be limited.

Turbinate Surgery

Reduction of a concha bullosa of the middle turbinate may be necessary, especially in the older child. The approach is the same as for the adult. A vertical incision is made into the anterior end of the turbinate, and the medial portion is preserved. Punch forceps or the microdebrider removes the lateral turbinate posterior to the hiatus semilunaris and medial bulla ethmoidalis, where the main areas of obstruction occur. Hemostasis is controlled with endoscopic cautery.

In general, middle turbinates in children should be preserved unless they are so diseased as to be part of the problem. Occasionally, a middle turbinate can be hypertrophic secondary to allergy or chronic rhinitis. Simple endoscopic anterior cautery with a needle-tipped unipolar cautery in cases where medical therapy has failed can be helpful. Usually there is not enough boggy, swollen mucosa to render the microdebrider useful, but occasionally the turbinate is polypoid and the microdebrider works nicely.

The inferior turbinates, when markedly hypertrophic and where medical treatment has failed, can be reduced with cautery, cryotherapy, or the powered microdebrider.[13] The removal of inferior turbinates in children is rarely necessary and should not be routinely done because of potential long-term problems. Cryotherapy in the author's hands has not been as successful as endoscopic submucosal cautery. The areas cauterized or microdebrided are usually limited to the anterior middle turbinates, where most edema is noted. The turbinate surgery is combined with turbinate outfracture to maximize the airway opening. The endoscopic microdebrider adequately removes edematous, inflamed turbinate

soft tissue. However, some bleeding is noted afterward, and light cautery or packing is required.

CHOANAL ATRESIA

Endoscopic visualization has greatly changed the ability to treat choanal atresia.[14] Powered instrumentation in the form of a microdrill has been used for a long time. The microdebrider adds the ability to handle the soft tissue with mucosal preservation and preciseness.[12] The smaller debrider tips (2.0–2.5 mm) are used. The approach consists of topical and injected analgesia placement followed by endoscopic evaluation. The incision is made in the mucosa overlying the atresia with a small Beaver blade or sickle knife. A cruciate incision can be made, as traditionally described, or superior- or inferior-based flaps can be made and elevated with a small elevator. Once bone is exposed, the microdrill is used medially toward the septum, making an opening on both sides. Drilling is then performed laterally. If the atresia is membranous, the microdebrider can create an opening and enlarge it as necessary. The vomerine part of the septum is removed with backward-biting forceps widely opening the atresia. Stents may or may not be necessary since mucosa has been preserved and raw surface is limited. A second-look procedure scheduled at 4–6 weeks may show some granulation and scarring, which can easily be debrided with the microdebrider to maintain the surgical opening.

ENDOSCOPIC SINUS SURGERY

Powered instrumentation in sinus surgery has been shown to be a valuable addition to the surgical armamentarium.[15,16] Gradually, powered instrumentation is becoming the workhorse of endoscopic sinus surgery. Along with through-cutting punch forceps, it provides the surgeon with the ability to perform targeted, functional endoscopic sinus surgery. When sinus surgery is necessary in the child, the initial surgery is directed at the anterior ethmoid and maxillary antrostomy, where most problems occur. The nose is prepared with a topical vasoconstrictor spray such as oxymetazoline. Cocaine is not contraindicated in the pediatric population, although some

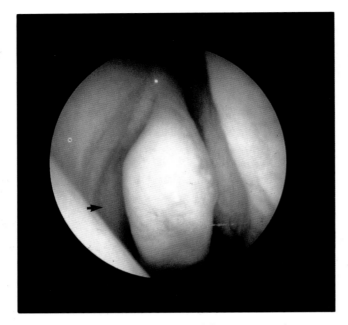

Figure 9.1. View of the right middle meatus and uncinate process (*arrow*).

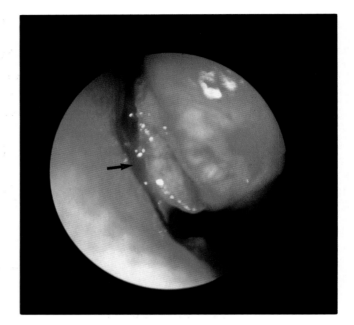

Figure 9.2. Incised uncinate process (*arrow*).

clinicians feel it should not be used. Pretreating with oxymetazoline reduces the systemic absorption of cocaine, decreasing any risk of complications. An alternative is to use a 1:10000 saline epinephrine solution topically. Xylocaine with epinephrine is injected to localize the nose.

The middle turbinate is preserved and gently pushed medially (Figure 9.1). If the septum is pushing the middle turbinate laterally, an endoscopic septoplasty can be performed to gain exposure. The uncinate process is incised with a sickle knife or cottle elevator. As an alternative, a small backward-biting forceps can be placed in the hiatus semilunaris, removing the uncinate from posterior to anterior (Figure 9.2). Small punch forceps or the microdebrider can release the uncinate, and the microdebrider can remove the uncinate (Figure 9.3). Where bone is too thick to be microdebrided, it can be removed with punch forceps and the soft tissue microdebrided. Often, after adequate removal of the uncinate, the maxillary antrostomy is found to be patent and the surgery is done (Figure 9.4). If not, the natural ostia is found by probing and dilated posteriorly. The antrostomy is opened posteriorly and inferiorly using the microdebrider or punch for-

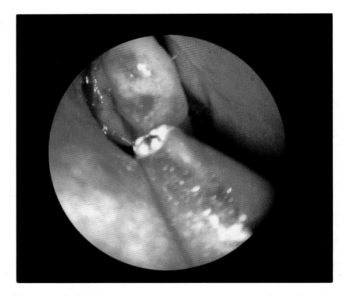

Figure 9.3. Uncinate process is removed with the microdebrider.

ceps (Figure 9.5). A punch forceps is used if bone is thickened posteriorly. A backward biter should not be used anteriorly due to the proximity of the nasolacrimal duct in children. At this point, if the CT scan or endoscopic examination does not demon-

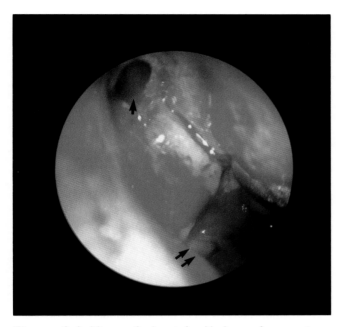

Figure 9.4. View of the infundibulum after uncinate process removal. Note the frontal recess (*arrow*) and patent antrostomy (*double arrow*).

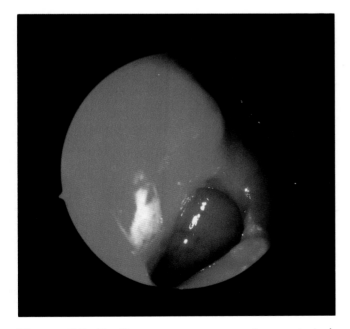

Figure 9.5. Maxillary antrostomy opening posteriorly using the microdebrider.

strate disease in the bulla or posterior ethmoid, the procedure is finished. Rolled Gelfilm or Telfa which does not cover the maxillary antrostomy is inserted. An alternative is to use a commercial stent, which can be removed after 3–4 weeks, or to suture the middle turbinate to the septum. An adhesion procedure whereby the middle turbinate and septum are scored opposite each other to produce local scarring can also be helpful but requires a small pack to be in place for 1–2 weeks.

In more extensive disease or if repeat surgery is necessary, the bulla is opened medially with a punch forceps and then removed with the microdebrider (Figure 9.6). The punch forceps is used to remove any thickened bone. The posterior ethmoids are approached through the basal lamella, which is always identified prior to entrance. Measurements of distances compared to a choanal measurement ensures proper localization. The basal lamella can be entered with punch forceps or the microdebrider (Figure 9.7). The basal lamella is removed and the posterior ethmoid inspected. Mucosal disease is removed with the microdebrider. The natural drainage opening of the posterior ethmoid is always checked for patency. This opening is found medially to the middle turbinate in the sphenoethmoidal recess. If the opening is blocked, it can easily be opened with the microdebrider, completing the ethmoidectomy (Figure 9.8).

The sphenoid sinus is rarely operated on in pediatric patients. However, if necessary, the sphenoid is approached through the ethmoid, medial to the middle turbinate, or, in the case of an isolated sphenoid infection, via partial removal of the lower portion of the middle turbinate, which approaches the sphenoid through the posterior ethmoid, preserving all the anterior sinuses.[17] The sphenoid opening is found with the aid of endoscopic visualization, measurement, and a probe. Computerized localization, if available, can be helpful. The superior turbinate may require partial removal, for which the microdebrider or small punch forceps is very helpful. Once the opening is found, it is gently dilated with a small, straight forceps. The microdebrider, working medially and laterally, can make an appropriate sphenoidotomy. Sphenoid punch forceps may also be helpful for further enlargement of the opening. Great care is taken to avoid opening the sinus inferi-

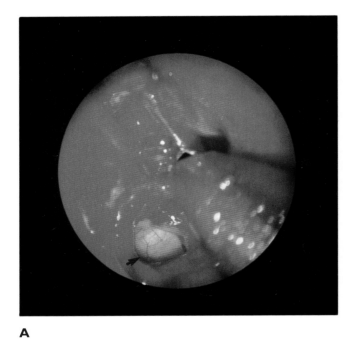

A

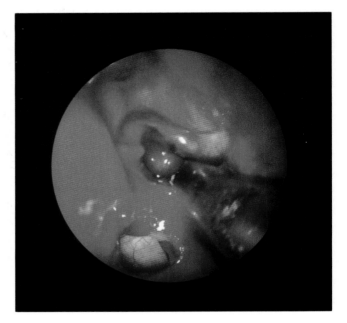

Figure 9.7. Basal lamella opened with the microdebrider.

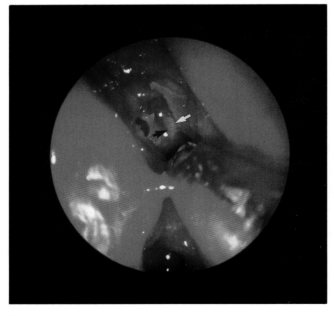

B

Figure 9.6. A: Bulla ethmoidalis is opened using the microdebrider. Note the antrostomy just anterior (*arrow*) to the bulla. **B:** Finished opening of the bulla ethmoidalis basal lamella (*arrow*) is visualized.

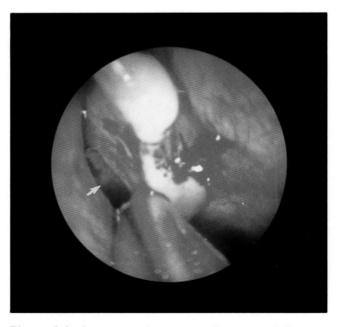

Figure 9.8. Superior turbinate partially removed. Opening to the posterior ethmoid drainage is enlarged with the microdebrider (*arrow*).

orly to prevent bleeding from the posterior septal artery. Prophylactic cautery in this area should be considered.

The frontal recess should not be violated in a child unless there is evidence of disease requiring attention. This will usually occur in the older child or teenager. Again, the uncinate process and agger nasi are opened with the microdebrider or small curved probes. Actual instrumentation of the frontal sinus should be avoided unless there is a good reason to do so.[18] Limited frontal recess anterior ethmoid surgery is often all that is necessary. If the frontal recess is opened, great care is taken postoperatively to avoid middle turbinate lateralization and scarring in the frontal recess. If only a small opening can be made in the frontal recess, a small 6 or 8 French feeding tube or suction catheter can be trimmed and used as a stent for 2–3 weeks postoperatively. Nothing is more frustrating and difficult to deal with than a child with recurrent frontal sinus problems after endoscopic sinus surgery.

Postoperative care in the child can be difficult, and a second-look procedure 3–4 weeks after the initial procedure should be planned in all children. If the child or young adult is very cooperative with postoperative packing removal and debridement, this exam can be canceled. However, if there is any concern for scarring or healing problems, it should be done. In one study, 50% of the maxillary antrostomies were closed or closing at the time of the second-look procedure.[2] Aggressive granulation was also noted. In some instances, a third-look procedure may be necessary to ensure proper healing.

COMPLICATIONS

Complications in pediatric endoscopic sinus surgery are rare.[2,19–21] No major complications, including orbital or brain injury, have been reported. The overall complication rate, excluding synechia, is less than 2%. Unfortunately, there is nothing in the literature regarding objective findings after endoscopic sinus surgery, so no comment can be made about delayed complications such as synechia. On the whole, however, children seem to do well with endoscopic sinus surgery. Some natural protection is afforded to children because the bone of the lam-

ina papyracea and skull base appear to be thickened during development and become more adult-like only as children approach the teenage years. Also, more experienced pediatric surgeons appear to be operating on children, lessening their overall risk. Long-term complications such as facial growth considerations will remain for the future. The addition of powered instrumentation to perform limited targeted endoscopic sinus surgery can only enhance safety and limit further complications.

CONCLUSION

Powered instrumentation enhances the endoscopic nasal and sinus surgeon's ability to remove disease precisely and conservatively in the pediatric population. Recognizing the differences between adults and children is important in applying the necessary instrumentation and skills to perform appropriate, safe sinus and nasal surgery in the pediatric population.

REFERENCES

1. Parsons DS, Setliff RC, Chambers DW: Special considerations in pediatric functional endoscopic sinus surgery. *Oper Tech Otolaryngol-Head Neck Surg* 5:40–42, 1994.
2. Stankiewicz JA: Pediatric endoscopic nasal and sinus surgery. *Otolaryngol Head Neck Surg* 113:204–210, 1995.
3. Krouse JH, Christmas DA: Powered instrumentation in functional endoscopic sinus surgery II: a comparative study. *ENT J.* 75(1):42–44, 1996.
4. Rosenfeld RM: Pilot study of outcomes in pediatric rhinosinusitis. *Arch Otolaryngol Head Neck Surg* 121(7):729–736, 1995.
5. Parsons DS: Chronic sinusitis. *Otolaryngol Clin North Am.* 29(1):1–9, 1996.
6. Mair EA, Bolger WE, Breisch EA: Sinus and facial growth after pediatric endoscopic sinus surgery. *Arch Otolaryngol Head Neck Surg* 121(5):547–552, 1995.
7. Otten FW, Aurem AV, Grote JJ: Long term follow-up of chronic maxillary sinusitis in children. *Int J Pediatr Otorhinolaryngol* 22:81–84, 1991.

8. Rachelefsky GS, Katz RM, Siegel SC: Chronic sinusitis in children with respiratory allergy. *J Allergy Clin Immunol* 69:382–387, 1982.

9. Ghandi A, Brodsky C, Ballow M: Benefits of prophylactic antibiotic prophylaxis in chronic sinusitis. *Allergy Pract* 14:37–43, 1993.

10. Borbero GJ: Gastroesophageal reflux and upper airway disease. *Otolaryngol Clin North Am* 29(1):27–38, 1996.

11. Vander Veken PJ, Clement PA, Bursseret T: Age related CT scan study of the incidence of sinusitis in children. *Am J Rhinol* 6:45–48, 1992.

12. Parsons DS: Rhinologic uses of powered instrumentation in children beyond sinus surgery. *Otolaryngol Clin North Am* 29(1):105–114, 1996.

13. Davis WE, Nishioka GJ: Endoscopic partial inferior turbinectomy using a power microcutting instrument. *ENT J* 75(1):49–50, 1996.

14. Stankiewicz JA: The endoscopic repair of choanal atresia. *Otolaryngol Head Neck Surg* 103:931–937, 1990.

15. Setliff RC: Minimally invasive sinus surgery: the rationale and technique. *Otolaryngol Clin North Am* 29(1):115–130, 1996.

16. Christmas DA, Krouse JH: Powered instrumentation in functional endoscopic sinus surgery I: surgical technique. *ENT J* 75(1):33–41, 1996.

17. Smith NC, Boyd EM: Pediatric sphenoidotomy. *Otolaryngol Clin North Am* 29(1):159–167, 1996.

18. Talbot AR: Frontal sinus surgery in children. *Otolaryngol Clin North Am* 29(1):143–157, 1996.

19. Parsons DS, Phillips D: Functional endoscopic sinus surgery in children: a retrospective analysis. *Laryngoscope* 103:899–903, 1993.

20. Gross CW, Gurucharri MJ, Lazar RH: Functional endoscopic sinus surgery (FESS) in the pediatric age group. *Laryngoscope* 99:272–275, 1989.

21. Lazar RH, Younis RT, Gross CW: Pediatric functional endonasal sinus surgery: review of 210 cases. *Head Neck Surg* 14:92–98, 1992.

10

Nursing Care of the Patient Undergoing Powered Endoscopic Sinus Surgery

Helene J. Krouse, Ph.D., R.N., C.S.

Nursing management of the patient undergoing functional endoscopic sinus surgery is a critical component in the overall success of treatment. In the office setting, the nurse acts as patient coordinator, organizing evaluation and diagnostic workup, patient teaching, and follow-up care. The knowledgeable nurse will be able to assist the patient through the health care system with ease, efficiency, and optimal outcome.

ASSESSMENT AND INITIAL EVALUATION

The individual with complaints of chronic sinus problems is often a prime candidate for sinus surgery. Initial evaluation of the patient in the office includes the patient's history of symptoms and treatments associated with the sinus problem. This history will include a discussion of the pattern of the symptoms, inciting and relieving factors, and prior use of medical and surgical interventions. In addition, the history will attempt to elicit any allergic component to the disease process, such as seasonality or known sensitivities. The physician will then perform a comprehensive head and neck examination, with special attention to the nasal cavity and nasopharynx for acute infections, inflammation, nasal polyps, and anatomic deformities that could compromise breathing. Definitive diagnosis of the extent of the sinus disease cannot be confirmed without a computed tomography (CT) scan and nasal endoscopy.[1,2]

During this initial evaluation, the patient will be scheduled for a CT scan in radiology. Generally a screening scan is performed, with a limited number of coronal views of the sinuses forming the evaluation. At times the physician may wish to obtain a more extensive CT study, with full coronal and axial views of the head. The patient will be given a second office appointment following the completion of the CT scan to review the results of the test with the physician. At this second visit, the patient will also undergo nasal endoscopy (Figure 10.1) and discuss available treatment options.

Many health insurance companies currently require precertification prior to scheduling the CT scan. It is important for the nurse to obtain this precertification in order to allow the patient to utilize his or her health insurance benefits for this often expensive study. In addition, precertification is often necessary for the office nasal endoscopy which is conducted at this follow-up appointment. The nurse can obtain precertification for both the CT scan and the office nasal endoscopy at this time. The CPT code used for billing office nasal endoscopy procedures is 31231.

The decision to offer the patient sinus surgery is determined by several factors. First a diagnosis of chronic sinusitis is substantiated through a positive

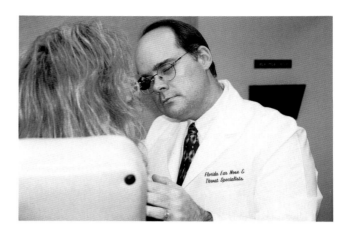

Figure 10.1. Nasal endoscopy.

patient history and confirming pathology on CT scan. In some cases, nasal endoscopic examination may suggest the utility of surgery even when the CT scan is equivocal. Quality of life issues are also considered in determining the appropriateness of a patient for surgical intervention such as days lost at work, altered lifestyle, and complaints of feeling badly most of the time. The purpose of powered endoscopic sinus surgery is reviewed along with its risks and benefits. It is important to provide the patient with realistic expectations of the surgical intervention. Allergy sufferers with significant chronic sinusitis will usually note improvement from their sinus problems with surgery, however, they will need to continue their allergy regimens postoperatively to maintain control of allergic symptoms and maximize treatment results.

Once the patient has decided to undergo powered endoscopic sinus surgery, the nurse must schedule the surgery, set up an appointment for the preoperative evaluation, and precertify the surgery with the patient's insurance company. At the time of surgical approval, certification for postoperative endoscopic debridement in the office should be confirmed. The CPT code for postoperative endoscopic debridement is 31237. The nurse should record this precertifica-

tion information on the surgical information sheet for quick reference as needed.

PREOPERATIVE EVALUATION

The role of the nurse during the preoperative evaluation is to prepare the patient for surgery. The nurse acts as preoperative coordinator of patient care by organizing the medical and diagnostic workup, providing preoperative instructions, scheduling surgery and related appointments, and answering questions.

The medical and diagnostic workup includes a thorough health history and physical examination. The nurse should obtain baseline data on vital signs and arrange for appropriate laboratory tests. Preparing a checklist of activities to complete prior to surgery will facilitate this task as preoperative coordinator and ensure that the patient is ready to proceed with the surgery. Preoperative preparation includes a complete medical history, blood work, routine diagnostic tests, and preoperative instructions. A preoperative checklist guide is provided to help organize the preoperative care and instruction (Appendix A).

Medication History

It is essential that the nurse obtains a complete medication history from the patient prior to the scheduled sinus surgery. The highly vascular nature of the tissue in the nasal and sinus cavities increases the likelihood of hemorrhage if proper bleeding precautions are not maintained. Patients should be screened for use of both prescriptive medications and over-the-counter remedies. Medications that increase bleeding time and disrupt coagulation include aspirin, nonsteroidal anti-inflammatory agents (e.g., ibuprofen), and anticoagulants (e.g., warfarin). These medications will have to be stopped for at least 1 week prior to surgery to restore normal clotting times. Patients who have been accustomed to taking these medications for other medical reasons need reassurance that a temporary cessation in their medication will not produce longstanding consequences.

Patients receiving long-term systemic steroids will need to be carefully monitored during the surgical procedure and postoperatively to prevent complications. This should be boldly noted on the chart along with medication allergies. In most cases, a burst dosage of intravenous steroids will be administered intraoperatively in these patients.

Diagnostic Testing

The nurse prepares all the paperwork and schedules appointments for laboratory and diagnostic tests. The nature of preoperative laboratory testing has been undergoing modification in recent years, with fewer studies generally being ordered. Routine testing at this point should include a complete blood count (CBC), bleeding time, prothrombin time (PT), and partial thromboplastin time (PTT). Chemistry profiles are appropriate in patients on certain cardiac medications or diuretics, and when felt to be appropriate in individual cases. The laboratory work needs to be done prior to surgery and results obtained before anesthesia is administered. The nurse should review these results prior to surgery to ensure that the patient has adequate clotting times and is not at an increased risk for bleeding. Other routine diagnostic tests include electrocardiogram and chest x-ray depending on the patient's age and health status.

Initial Preparation for Surgery

Patients also receive instructions by the nurse for the day of surgery. The patient is advised to not eat or drink anything after midnight. Important medications can be taken in the early morning on arising with a very small sip of water. Patients must arrange a ride home from the office, ambulatory facility, or hospital after the procedure, as they will not be allowed to drive home due to the anesthetic or sedation. Providing patients with a written checklist in preparation for their surgery will be very beneficial. These materials include reminders to avoid medications with aspirin and aspirin-containing products.

Patients should also be told to complete laboratory work 48 h before the scheduled surgery. In most cases, the patient can be scheduled for a preoperative appointment at the hospital or outpatient surgical facility in order to assure adequate time to receive and review all results. A phone call by the nurse just prior to the day of surgery will be very reassuring to the patient and family. The nurse will have an opportunity to remind the patient of the specific date and time of the procedure and review preoperative instructions as needed. This phone contact also allows the patient an opportunity to ask questions, receive clarifications, or allay any anxieties that may have arisen since the preoperative evaluation in the office.

PATIENT TEACHING

A major role of the nurse preoperatively and postoperatively is to educate the patient regarding perioperative care (Figure 10.2). Patient teaching should be initiated at the time the patient elects to undergo surgery and proceeds throughout follow-up care. A major goal of preoperative instruction is to alleviate patient anxiety by preparing for what is to happen and how to facilitate recovery from surgery with optimal results.

Patients can prepare for the postoperative period by filling their prescriptions for pain medication and antibiotics prior to surgery. This policy of providing prescriptions prior to surgery helps the patients to feel more in control of their care. It also avoids the

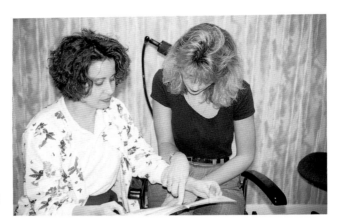

Figure 10.2. Patient instruction regarding surgery.

inconvenience of having a family member stop at a pharmacy to purchase these medications during the immediate postoperative period. Many patients are concerned about postoperative pain and feel relieved knowing that they have a medication on hand to alleviate these symptoms. Patients who do not wish to use prescriptive pain medications can find good relief with acetaminophen.

Reducing the Chance of Bleeding

The nurse should also briefly discuss measures to promote healing and reduce the common complications of infection and mild postoperative bleeding. A written instruction sheet is provided for enhancing patient teaching and is reviewed both preoperatively and postoperatively with the patient. Specific measures to employ to reduce the chances of postoperative bleeding include the avoidance of nose blowing, coughing or sneezing with mouth open, and avoiding aspirin and nonsteroidal anti-inflammatory medications.

Patients initiate use of phenylephrine ½% or oxymetazoline 0.05% sprays immediately after surgery. The spray is to be used one or two sprays in each operated nostril, three times a day for 3 days,

then thereafter only if the nose bleeds. If bleeding is persistent, the patient is instructed to spray a tissue and insert a portion of it into the nostril to stop the bleeding.

Patients are also instructed to limit their physical activities. Restrictions on activities include avoiding bending, lifting, straining, strenuous activities, and exercise.[3] The patient is instructed to avoid extremes in temperature such as direct sun and extremely cold weather. Travel is limited to the nearby area until the surgeon has cleared the patient. Changes in altitude and pressure associated with airplane travel can result in increases in blood pressure and predispose the patient to bleeding.

Patients should also be informed of postoperatively bleeding from the nose that will occur within the first few days at home. They should be told that some bleeding from the nose is to be expected but will slow down over the first 48 h and usually subsides completely within 3–4 days. If significant bleeding occurs, the patient is instructed to spit the blood out rather than swallow the blood to reduce chances of becoming nauseated and vomiting.

Bleeding may be further reduced by keeping the head elevated and by applying ice bags. Some individuals find it most comfortable to sleep with their head elevated on several pillows or on a recliner for the first 24–48 h after surgery. Elevating the head will decrease bleeding and promote comfort by helping to drain the area and relieving pressure. Applying ice bags near the nose and cheeks may also be helpful in reducing bleeding and swelling in the area.[3]

The patient is instructed to call the office if heavy bleeding is noted. Should the patient call to report significant bleeding, it is important to advise the patient to describe the amount of bleeding he or she is experiencing in order to determine the severity. Heavy bleeding may require further intervention by the physician to control it.

Promoting Healing

During surgery the patient will receive a bolus dose of antibiotics to help reduce the chances of infections postoperatively. Many otolaryngologists also start patients on a course of antibiotic therapy postoperatively for 5 to 10 days. Various medications are used postoperatively, and may involve a penicillin or cephalosporin. Clindamycin is an effective alternative medication in the case of allergies to penicillins and cephalosporins.

Some physicians also initiate antibiotic ointments such as gentamicin sulfate 0.1%. This ointment is directly squeezed into the nostril from the tube in the morning and at bedtime (Figure 10.3). The patient should be clearly instructed not to stick fingers or blunt objects directly into the nose to insert the ointment. Scratching or ripping this sensitive area will greatly increase the chances of infection and bleeding.

Some patients receive relief from nasal congestion, stuffiness, and headaches by using a humidifier in the room. Keeping the nostrils moist will prevent crusting. If the nose is not packed, patients begin using saline sprays. The patient is instructed to use three to four squirts in each nostril every 1 to 2 h while awake. The patient occludes the opposite nostril and breathes in while spraying. Patients continue with these saline sprays for 3 to 4 weeks postoperatively to keep the membranes moist and reduce crusting and bleeding.

In addition, patients usually begin a nasal steroid spray such as beclomethasone at their first postoperative visit. These sprays decrease nasal edema in the postoperative period, and are of great importance in patients with significant nasal polyposis as part of an indefinite treatment strategy.

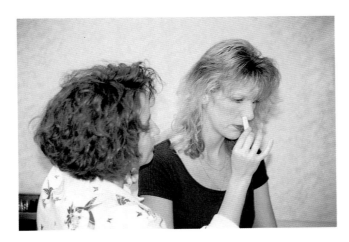

Figure 10.3. Applying antibiotic ointment into nostril.

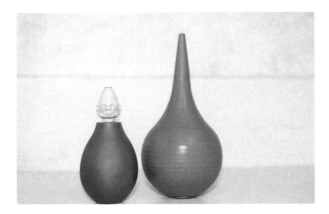

Figure 10.4. Syringes for nasal irrigation.

Nasal Irrigation

In addition to nasal saline sprays, many otolaryngologists recommend nasal irrigations after the first postoperative visit. Nasal irrigations wash out the nasal cavity, cleanse the nose, and control accumulation of crusting by washing with a stream of water.[4] These irrigations also liquefy secretions and

improve mucociliary clearance.[5] The irrigation solution can be made by mixing the following ingredients:

1 quart water (boiled)
1 teaspoon salt
1 teaspoon of baking soda

The patient can prepare extra solution and keep the unused portion in the refrigerator. The irrigation solution should be at room temperature before irrigating the nose.[3] Excessive heat will increase chances of bleeding, therefore a cooler irrigant is recommended rather than a warmer solution.

A nasal syringe or bulb syringe may be used to irrigate the nose (Figure 10.4). A nasal syringe has a wide, blunt tip that allows the patient to insert only a limited length of the syringe into the nasal cavity. The bulb syringe is often used in ear irrigations and has a much longer and narrower shaft. The patient is instructed to insert the tip of the syringe only ¾ to 1 inch into the nostril (Figure 10.5).

The patient irrigates each operated nostril with one cup of saline solution by first squeezing the syringe in the solution to fill it (Figure 10.6). The patient leans over a sink and inserts the syringe in the nostril. With a firm squeeze on the bulb, the patient irrigates the nostril (Figure 10.7). The solu-

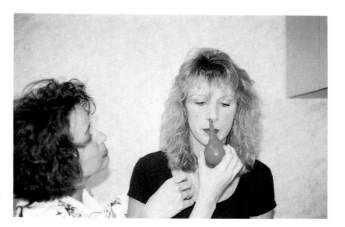

Figure 10.5. Irrigating tip inserted into nostril.

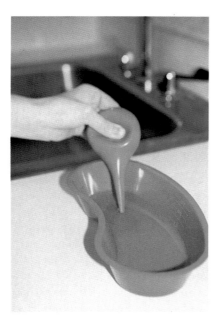

Figure 10.6. Drawing saline solution into bulb syringe.

tion should enter one nostril and drain out of the other side. The patient repeats this procedure until the solution is finished, and then follows the same irrigation procedure on the opposite side if bilateral surgery was performed.

The patient optimally will perform this nasal irrigation three times a day to properly cleanse the area and reduce crusting and bleeding. The nurse must encourage the patient to develop comfort in the procedure through careful instruction in the technique. Damage can be done to the nose if the patient inserts the tip too far or is overly aggressive in irrigating the nose. This same saline solution can also be placed in a spray bottle and used as a nasal spray as well as an irrigant.

Proper patient education is critical to the overall success of the surgical procedure. The nurse must be sure to allow ample time to instruct patients, encourage questions and elicit feedback on materials presented, and provide supplemental written materials to further reinforce teaching. An example of areas to include in the preoperative instruction for patients is included in Appendix A.

Diet and Fluid Intake

Patients are instructed also on the importance of following some dietary limitations in the immediate postoperative period. They are encouraged to maintain good hydration in the first few days after surgery, and told that it is not essential to begin intake of solid foods at this time. Immediately on

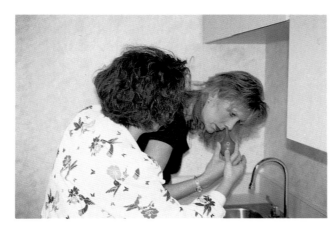

Figure 10.7. Irrigating nose over sink.

arriving home from surgery a full liquid diet is appropriate, with a gradual progression to a regular diet as tolerated. Patients are advised to avoid hot foods and liquids, as they can increase bleeding through their vasodilatory effects.

POSTOPERATIVE CARE

Postoperative Assessment

Nursing assessment in the postoperative period focuses on several areas, including bleeding, facial swelling and ecchymosis, pain, hydration, and fluid tolerance. Some mild bleeding is expected in the immediate postoperative period, and might continue for several days. Profuse bleeding or hemorrhage is not common, however, and is cause for concern. The nurse monitors the amount of bleeding during the time spent in the surgical facility, looking for signs of significant bleeding into the throat, frequent changing of the drip pad taped under the nose, or changes in vital signs. Patients are advised to observe the amount of bleeding upon discharge home, and to notify the office for any significant increase in the quantity of bleeding at home. The nurse can be of assistance in reinforcing preoperative teaching at this time, offering the patient guidance and reassurance.

An unusual but severe complication in powered endoscopic sinus surgery is orbital hemorrhage. In this situation significant bleeding occurs in the orbit itself, causing a significant increase in intraocular pressure. If not treated quickly, blindness can result. The earliest signs of orbital bleeding are periorbital ecchymosis and swelling of the eye. These are emergency situations, and the physician must be notified immediately. While this bleeding can be brisk and lead to rapid swelling and bruising, at times it can occur more gradually over the first 24 to 48 hr. For this reason, patients are advised to notify the office if any signs of facial ecchymosis or swelling of the eyes or eyelids occurs.

Postoperative assessment also is important to evaluate for signs of changes in mental status, neck stiffness, confusion, or unusual sedation. Injury to the cribriform plate or other areas of the skull base can occur during sinus surgery, and any neurologic findings or symptoms and signs suggestive of meningitis are important. Again, these mental status changes can be observed in the early postoperative period, or can develop over the first several days at home. Patients and families are counseled in these possible consequences, and advised to report any suspicious symptoms.

Postoperative pain is usually mild following powered endoscopic sinus surgery, but can be somewhat more severe if a concurrent nasal septoplasty or rhinoplasty has been performed. The most frequent cause of significant discomfort following nasal surgery is the use of nasal packing. Nasal packing, however, is rarely necessary after sinus surgery unless additional nasal surgery has been completed. Narcotic pain medications are usually prescribed postoperatively, and can be of greatest use at bedtime. The need for narcotic analgesia abates rapidly after surgery, and after the removal of nasal packing if used. The nurse can be of assistance in counseling patients regarding the appropriate use of pain medications following surgery, and in assessing any unusual requirements for analgesia.

In most cases of nasal and sinus surgery, the patient swallows some blood intraoperatively and immediately following surgery. Blood is especially irritative to the stomach, and often provokes nausea and some vomiting during the first 24 hr. While some vomiting is common, persistent vomiting is of concern as it will affect fluid hydration and electrolyte balance. The nurse in the surgical setting must assess the amount of fluid intake and the absence of significant vomiting prior to discharge. In addition, the patient must be advised to continue good fluid hydration at home, and to report any significant vomiting, especially gross hematemesis. Again, reassurance and reference to the preoperative teaching protocol can be quite helpful here.

Postoperative Follow-up Care

The nurse should contact the patient by phone the afternoon of discharge to inquire about how he or she is doing at home, and to ask if there are any questions which the family might have at this point.

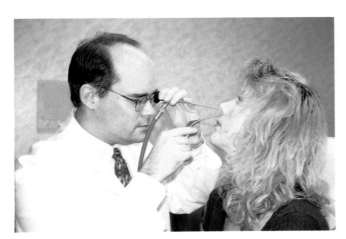

Figure 10.8. Postoperative nasal debridement.

This personal contact is of great benefit in assuring patients that the surgical team is aware of their condition and available for assistance if necessary. Patients are also reminded of the follow-up appointment, which had been previously scheduled at the preoperative session, and to contact the office if any problems occur.

The patient is generally seen back in the office at 2 to 4 days after surgery. At that time the nasal cavity is evaluated and debrided endoscopically (Figure 10.8). Issues such as postoperative bleeding and hydration are critical at this first visit. The nurse will spend a significant time at this visit as well on the topics of nasal irrigation, the use of nasal sprays and ointments, and issues of diet and return to activity. In addition, the nurse can inquire into any specific problems which the patient may be encountering at home, and develop strategies for dealing with those individual problems.

Follow-up visits continue regularly over the first 6 to 8 weeks following surgery, and generally taper back from weekly visits initially. At each of these visits, the nurse has the opportunity to reassess the patient's progress, to offer reassurance and reinforcement, and to answer any specific questions which may arise.

CONCLUSION

The otolaryngology nurse plays an integral role in the management of the patient undergoing powered endoscopic sinus surgery. Through the nurse's role as patient educator and advocate, the patient is instructed in specific skills and techniques which encourage postoperative healing and facilitate patient compliance with treatment. The nurse's intervention decreases patient anxiety around the time of surgery, and offers reassurance and support following the operative procedure. In addition, the nurse's clinical expertise in assisting the patient through the preoperative workup maximizes the safety of the surgery. All of these functions of the otolaryngology nurse contribute to a surgical experience for the patient which maximizes treatment outcomes and reduces patient anxiety and apprehension.

REFERENCES

1. Kennedy DW, Kennedy EM: Endoscopic sinus surgery. *AORN J* 42:932–936, 1985.
2. Thawley SE, Garrett H: Endoscopic sinus surgery:

an outpatient procedure that minimizes tissue removal. *AORN J* 47:890–897, 1988.
3. Sigler BA, Schuring LT: *Ear, Nose, and Throat Disorders.* St Louis, Mosby, 1993.
4. Riley MA: *Nursing Care of the Client with Ear, Nose, and Throat Disorders.* New York, Springer, 1987.
5. Schwartz R: The diagnosis and management of sinusitis. *Nurse Practitioner* 19:58–63, 1994.

Appendix A

PATIENT PREOPERATIVE CHECKLIST

- Eliminate aspirin-containing medications, and nonsteroidal anti-inflammatory medications (such as ibuprofen) 2 weeks before surgery
- Tell your doctor about any medications you are taking, especially any recently prescribed medications
- Do not eat or drink anything after midnight the night before surgery
- Ask your doctor whether you should take any of your regular medications the morning of surgery
- Arrange for a ride home after the operation
- Plan for preoperative laboratory testing 2 to 3 days prior to surgery
- Buy a bulb syringe for postoperative salt water irrigations of the nose
- Fill your prescriptions prior to surgery so the medications are on hand when you arrive home

Appendix B

HOME CARE AFTER POWERED ENDOSCOPIC SINUS SURGERY

What to Do and Expect After Surgery

1. Rest quietly for 48 hours after leaving the hospital. Keeping your head elevated on several pillows or using a recliner will decrease bleeding and pressure.

2. Ice bags placed near the nose over the cheeks may be helpful for the first 24 to 48 hours as tolerated.

3. If you have to sneeze or cough, keep your mouth open so you won't build up pressure in your nose. Don't suppress the need to sneeze or cough. To help minimize sneezing, you may use Benadryl 25 mg every 6 hours if needed.

4. Do not blow your nose until you have been given permission to do so.

5. Expect facial discomfort or headache. You have been given prescriptions for pain medications. Use these if needed as directed. Do not use aspirin or nonsteroidal anti-inflammatory medications (such as Advil, Nuprin, or Motrin).

6. Expect a dry and somewhat sore throat. Mouth breathing contributes to this feeling. Taking frequent liquids will help ease this sore throat.

7. Expect a low-grade fever. Do not use aspirin. For fever use Tylenol as needed and drink plenty of fluids. If your temperature goes above 102° F, call the office.

Bleeding

Expect bleeding from the nose and some down into your throat. Do not swallow the blood. Spit it out. If blood is swallowed, nausea and vomiting will result in most patients. Bleeding usually slows down over 48 hours. If bleeding persists, continue to use ice bags and keep your head elevated. Anxiety will increase the bleeding, so try to relax.

If a lot of bleeding persists after 48 hours, call the office. You may use a gauze pad under the nose to absorb the blood and discharge. Remove this gauze pad while eating or drinking, and replace it when you are finished.

Expect a lot of discolored drainage after the bleeding slows down. This will continue for at least several weeks.

Restrictions on Activity

Avoid bending, lifting, or straining.

Avoid strenuous activity and exercise until healing is completed.

Avoid extreme heat or cold. Stay out of the sun.

Avoid aspirin and aspirin-containing products.
Avoid travel out of your home area until healing is completed.

Diet

Eat a light diet over the first few days following surgery. Drink plenty of fluids. Many patients experience some nausea and vomiting after a general anesthetic. If this occurs, restrict yourself to fluids for 24–48 hours. If nausea or vomiting occurs longer than 24–48 hours, call the office.

Medications

Most patients are given medications for the following:

An *antibiotic*—Use as directed until the prescription is finished.

For *pain*—Use as directed, only if needed. You may use Tylenol also Do not use aspirin, aspirin-containing products or nonsteroidal anti-inflammatory medications.

For *fever*—Do not use aspirin! Use Tylenol if needed.

For *constipation*—Use a stool softener and mild laxative as needed to avoid straining.

Nasal Irrigations

Begin irrigating the nose when instructed to do so by the physician, using the separate instructions for nasal irrigations.

Call Us If You Have Any of the Following

- Temperature of over 102° F
- Visual problems or swelling or bulging of the eyes
- Neck stiffness with headache and fever
- Excessive drowsiness or confusion
- Profuse nosebleed you can't control

11

Postoperative Care and Follow-Up of the Surgical Site

Eiji Yanagisawa, M.D., F.A.C.S.
Dewey A. Christmas, Jr., M.D.
John H. Krouse, M.D., Ph.D., F.A.C.S.

INTRODUCTION

Patients who undergo powered endoscopic sinus surgery typically are discharged home on the day of the procedure after being observed in the ambulatory setting for several hours. These patients do not routinely have nasal packing unless extensive concurrent septal work has been performed or there has been excessive bleeding during the procedure. If inferior turbinate surgery is done at the same time as sinus surgery, some surgeons will place nasal packing as well. Most patients do have middle meatal stents placed at the time of surgery, which are removed in several weeks if not spontaneously extruded prior to that time.

Patients are discharged home with antibiotic medication to prevent infection, with narcotic analgesia, and sometimes with antinausea medications. In addition, they have previously received extensive education from the office nurse and physician regarding home care, instructions on activity, diet, limitations, and signs and symptoms for which they should alert the office.[1] They are given a follow-up appointment, generally at 24 to 48 hours following surgery.

FIRST POSTOPERATIVE VISIT (24–48 HOURS)

At this first visit following surgery, any nasal packing placed at the time of the procedure is removed

from the nasal cavity. There is usually some mild bleeding at this time, which generally stops quickly with some light pressure. The nose is then sprayed with a vasoconstricting agent such as phenylephrine 1% or ephedrine 3% solution. In addition, the nasal cavity is sprayed with a topical anesthetic such as xylocaine 2% or tetracaine 2% solution. These sprays shrink the nasal and turbinate mucosa, which is often edematous following surgery, to slow any oozing of blood and to provide a level of topical anesthesia for examination and cleaning of the cavities. Application of these topical agents is aided by spreading the nostrils with a nasal speculum. Generally, 5 minutes are then allowed for these medications to take effect.

At this point, anterior rhinoscopy is undertaken. The anterior nasal cavity is inspected for any bleeding sites, which can be cauterized if necessary with silver nitrate ($AgNO_3$). In addition, if septal surgery had been performed, the septum can be examined for signs of perforation, hematoma, or abscess. Any mucoid or clotted material can be suctioned clear at this time.

Instruments useful for postoperative care of powered endoscopic sinus surgery (PESS) patients are shown in Figure 11.1. These instruments include (1) 4-mm 0° telescope, (2) Frazier nasal suction tube (Fr. 10, 12), (3) right-angled suction tube, (4) long nasal cup or alligator forceps, (5) Hartmann ear forceps, and (6) right-angled ear hook. If nasal crusts are fixed, or are mobile and difficult to grasp, the use of a right-angled ear hook may be useful.

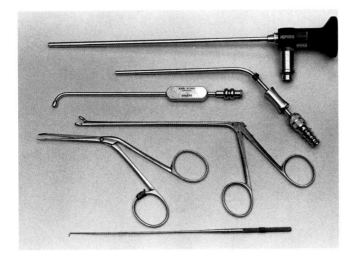

Figure 11.1. Instruments useful for postoperative PESS patients. Top to bottom: (1) 4-mm 0° telescope; (2) Frazier nasal suction tube; (3) right-angled nasal suction tube; (4) nasal cup or alligator forceps; (5) Hartmann ear forceps; (6) right-angled ear hook.

Nasal endoscopy is then carried out to evaluate the more posterior nares and to examine the middle meatus. At this point, Gelfilm stents are usually in position, so the entire middle meatus cannot be visualized. Stents are properly placed into the resected ethmoid system intraoperatively, taking care to avoid occlusion of the middle meatal maxillary antrostomy or natural ostium inferior to this area. The maxillary ostium can therefore be easily examined endoscopically and debrided of any mucoid material, crusting, or granulation tissue, even with the stents in place. These stents will be left in position for about 2 weeks but may be extruded prior to that time. Patients should be advised that these stents may be expelled spontaneously and will have the appearance of a wet soft contact lens. They can be instructed that if these stents do come out, no intervention is necessary and it is not a cause for concern.

Once the nasal cavity is cleaned, debrided, and thoroughly examined, patients receive a review of their home care instructions. At this time, they are advised to start on nasal irrigations in order to keep the cavity clean, rinse any mucoid or bloody material, and enhance mucociliary clearance. They have

been previously given an extensive postoperative instruction booklet,[1] which is reviewed at this time, and any instructions that are not understood by the patient are clarified by the physician and/or nurse. Patients are instructed in the hourly use of nasal saline spray and in the twice daily application of gentamicin sulfate 0.5% ophthalmic ointment (or Neomycin or Bacitracin ointment) into the nasal cavity to prevent infection and provide some lubrication. In addition, topical nasal corticosteroid sprays such as beclomethasone can be instituted or resumed at this time. Patients are discharged home from the office, to return again in 1 week.

SECOND POSTOPERATIVE VISIT (1 WEEK)

At the second visit, the physician and nurse review the patient's progress over the preceding week. Any significant problems, such as persistent bleeding, excessive pain, or nasal airway obstruction are discussed. The nose is then topically decongested and anesthetized once again, and anterior rhinoscopy is completed. In patients who have had inferior turbinate surgery there will likely be extensive crusting of the turbinate edge, which will continue for 4 to 6 weeks. Crusts which are easily removed can be cleared at this time, but vigorous debridement of these crusts will likely produce significant bleeding and should be avoided. The healing of the septal incision site can also be checked and the status of the mucoperichondrial flaps evaluated.

Nasal endoscopy can then be easily performed. The posterior nares can be visualized back to the nasopharynx and cleaned and debrided as necessary. If a transnasal sphenoidotomy was performed, the sphenoid ostium can be visualized; it may or may not be stented at this time. Attention is then paid to the middle meatus, where again the stents are usually still in position. Reepithelialization of the mucosa is generally rapid with the use of the microdebrider, and evidence of healing will be present at this 1-week visit. Again, any crusting or occlusion of the maxillary ostium can be debrided endoscopically at this time. Postoperative instructions are again reviewed with the patient, and the patient is discharged home to return again in 1 week.

THIRD POSTOPERATIVE VISIT (2 WEEKS)

At this time, the patient should be relatively symptom free, with no bleeding or significant discomfort. There may still be some residual nasal airway obstruction due to postoperative edema and turbinate crusting, especially if the laser was used for the turbinate surgery. Again, topical vasoconstricting agents and anesthetic sprays are applied to the nasal mucosa. By anterior rhinoscopy, any debridement of the anterior nasal cavity can be carried out at this time.

Nasal endoscopic examination is then completed. If any stents that were placed intraoperatively have not yet extruded, they should be removed by the surgeon at this time. These stents can be easily grasped with a bayonet or Blakesly forceps and removed. Often, crusts and some granulation tissue adherent to the stents are removed along with the stents. Once the stents are removed, an excellent examination of the prior ethmoidectomy is possible (Figure 11.2A). Any granulation tissue or scarring which is present can be easily debrided at this time. Usually, a nicely open surgical site is seen after the stents are

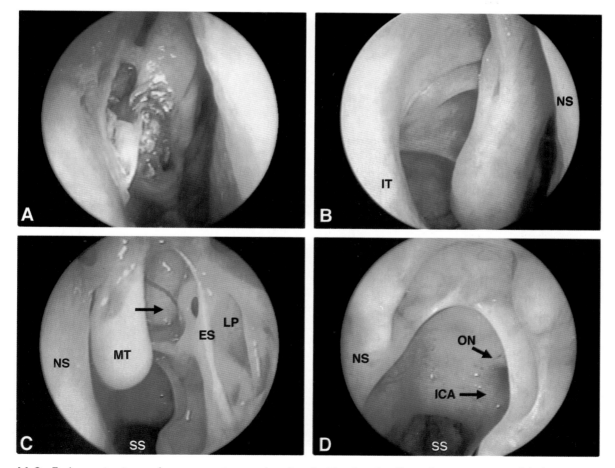

Figure 11.2. Endoscopic views of postoperative nasal cavity. **A:** Nasal cavity (2 weeks postoperatively) showing crusts covering the right middle turbinate. **B:** Nasal cavity (4 months postoperatively) showing a well-healed patent middle meatal antrostomy. **C:** Well-healed left sphenoethmoidectomy cavity (6 months postoperatively) showing the roof of the posterior ethmoid sinus (*arrow*). Note the vessel crossing the skull base. LP, lamina papyracea; ES, scarred tissues of the ethmoid sinus; MT, middle turbinate; NS, nasal septum; large sphenoidotomy opening. **D:** Well-healed sphenoethmoidectomy cavity (6 months postoperatively) showing a large sphenoid sinus opening (SS), optic nerve (ON), and internal carotid artery (ICA). Note the red spot just above the optic nerve caused by a suction tip.

removed. Sphenoid ostial stents are also removed at this visit if they are still in position. The sphenoid ostium can be similarly debrided and cleaned if necessary. A nicely patent sphenoidotomy is generally appreciated upon removal of the stents.

The general appearance of the sinus surgical sites at this 2-week visit is excellent. The epithelial regrowth is typically well underway, and crusting is usually minimal. The nasal airway is quite good. The patient is usually released to perform all routine activities at this time, unless there has been significant, persistent bleeding in the preceding week. The patient is instructed to continue nasal irrigations, saline spray, and ointment use and to return to the office in 2 weeks.

FOURTH POSTOPERATIVE VISIT (4 WEEKS)

By the time of this fourth visit, the sinus surgical sites have generally healed totally when powered instrumentation is utilized. The ability of this technology to preserve normal mucosa and to remove tissue with minimal trauma enhances the healing of the surgical areas through limited epithelial stripping. Since crusting is significantly reduced, postoperative granulation tissue is generally minimal, and complete epithelialization is usually noted by 4 weeks.

At this visit, the nasal cavity is again sprayed with topical anesthetic and vasoconstricting agents. Anterior rhinoscopy is used to clean the nares. Turbinate crusting is generally abating at this point, although it may still be present over the next several weeks. The posterior nares and sinuses are then examined with the nasal endoscope. At this time, very little cleaning or debridement is necessary in most cases. A nicely open maxillary antrostomy is appreciated, without stenosis and with epithelial covering of its edges circumferentially. The ethmoid sinuses are open, and the resection site has epithelialized quite well. The frontal recess can be well seen and is free of crusting or disease. The sphenoidotomy has also healed quite well, and its ostium is widely patent.

At this time, the patient can generally discontinue the use of nasal irrigations and rinses, and the surgical sites are well healed. In cases in which significant crusting does persist, rinses will be continued and the patient brought back at biweekly intervals until all crusting has ceased. Generally, this level of crusting is seen only in inferior turbinate surgery, although at times there can be more extensive crusting in the sinus areas as well. Regular follow-up will be maintained in these patients. Once all crusting has ceased in the postoperative period, a nicely healed surgical site can be appreciated (Figure 11.2B). The patient can then be discharged to extended follow-up, usually in 6 months.

EXTENDED FOLLOW-UP

Patients are generally brought back to the office at 6- to 12-month intervals following surgery. In cases of sinonasal polyposis, inverted papilloma, and allergic fungal sinusitis, lifetime follow-up is indicated due to the high likelihood of these processes to recur. Nasal endoscopy is performed at each follow-up visit to examine for recurrent polypoid disease or papilloma, recurrent infection, or other signs of persistent or recurrent disease. Cleaning and debridement of the surgical sites is performed quite easily in these patients, and biopsy or sampling of tissue is possible if indicated at this time.

In most cases, the appearance of the sites is quite good at extended follow-up. The maxillary ostium is generally nicely open, as is the sphenoid ostium. The ethmoid system is clear of disease. The frontal recess remains open and free of edema or infection. The general extended appearance of the surgical sites in powered endoscopic sinus surgery reflects well-healed mucosal surfaces with no inflammatory change.

When the sinus cavity is cleaned postoperatively with a suction tip or a pointed forceps, these instruments should be used gently and cautiously to prevent accidental injury to exposed vital structures such as anterior and posterior ethmoid vessels, the roof of the ethmoid sinuses, lamina papyracea, optic nerve, or internal carotid artery (Figure 11.2C, D).

REFERENCE

1. Krouse HJ: Nursing care of the patient undergoing powered endoscopic sinus surgery. In Krouse JH,

Christmas DA (eds): *Powered Endoscopic Sinus Surgery*. Baltimore, Williams & Wilkins, 1997, pp .

BIBLIOGRAPHY

Stammberger H: *Functional Endoscopic Sinus Surgery—The Messerklinger technique*. Philadelphia, Decker, 1991, pp 369–379.

Yanagisawa E, Yanagisawa K: Endoscopic view of exposed vital structures following sphenoethmoidectomy. *Ear Nose Throat J* 73:810–811, 1994.

Yanagisawa E, Yanagisawa K: Intranasal crusting following endoscopic surgery. *ENT J* 74:392–394, 1995.

12

Complications of Powered Endoscopic Sinus Surgery and Their Management

John H. Krouse, M.D., Ph.D., F.A.C.S.
James A. Stankiewicz, M.D., F.A.C.S.

As all surgeons appreciate, any operative procedure is accompanied by the risk of complications. In sinus surgery specifically, when complications do occur, they can be especially morbid or even fatal due to the proximity of the paranasal sinuses to critical anatomic structures in the head. Blindness, diplopia, serious hemorrhage, meningitis, brain injury, and even death have been reported subsequent to endoscopic sinus procedures. It is essential, therefore, for those physicians who practice endoscopic sinus surgery to take precautions to minimize the risk of these serious operative consequences, and to prepare themselves to deal with these profound events if and when they do occur.

BACKGROUND

Preoperative Training

It is well known that the experience of the surgeon directly affects the incidence of major complications in functional endoscopic sinus surgery.[1–3] As surgeons gain facility and comfort with endoscopic procedures, they are less likely to encounter serious complications. The first step in developing this experience must be to gain a thorough understanding of the surgical anatomy of the lateral nasal wall and paranasal sinuses. Once the surgeon achieves mastery of this difficult anatomy, it is important to develop facility with its endoscopic appearance in a cadaver laboratory. Also, in this laboratory setting, the otolaryngologist can begin to utilize the various surgical instruments on cadaver specimens. Through this thorough preparation in the academic and practical aspects of sinus surgery, the physician can begin to develop confidence and security with this often difficult surgical field.

Only when the otolaryngologist has achieved a sufficient level of comfort and skill in the laboratory setting can he or she begin to transfer this knowledge to the operating room setting on live patients. Powered devices should be used first on patients with mild polyposis and limited disease, and more difficult surgery attempted only after the surgeon feels comfortable with these more straightforward conditions. Surgeons with limited endoscopic surgical experience must proceed more gradually in order to gain facility with the endoscopes in addition to the powered devices. These otolaryngologists should begin with frequent use of the endoscopes in the office setting to acquire facility with their use and an appreciation of the intranasal anatomy.

Patient Evaluation

In order to minimize the risk of complications, it is important to evaluate each patient thoroughly prior to entering the operating room. The surgeon must be aware of any concurrent medical illnesses which might affect the patient's perioperative course. A history of prior nasal and sinus surgery is significant in that important landmarks can be obscured or absent in patients with previous operations. A history of abnormal bleeding from surgery or injuries suggests that a disorder of clotting may be present and directs further evaluation. In addition, a thorough medication history is essential, since patients taking aspirin or nonsteroidal anti-inflammatory medications will have a higher likelihood of significant intraoperative bleeding.

The patient's computed tomography (CT) scan must be evaluated both prior to surgery and in the operating room. The critical surgical anatomy must be visualized on the scan in order to minimize the likelihood of a serious injury to an important structure. The surgeon must identify the lamina papyracea and trace it back posteriorly toward the apex of the orbit. In addition, it is critical to note the depth of the olfactory fossa, recognizing that the most common site of intracranial penetration is medial, at the lateral lamella of the cribriform plate. With increasing depth of this fossa, there is a higher likelihood of medial penetration, as a larger area of thin bone is present medially. In addition, any bone dehiscences in the base of the skull should be noted on the CT scan, and any soft tissue masses which might be protruding into the sinuses superiorly will dictate further diagnostic workup prior to surgery.

In addition, thorough nasal endoscopy must be carried out in the office prior to bringing the patient to the operating room. Attention must be given to the patient's specific intranasal anatomy, and any unusual variations must be appreciated and noted prior to surgery. In addition, the surgeon can decide whether septal work is necessary in order to gain access to the middle meatus, and whether such a procedure should be completed at the time of the sinus surgery or staged.

Intraoperative Considerations

As noted above, the CT scan must be present in the operating room throughout the surgical procedure.

The scan serves as a "road map" for the procedure, and the skillful surgeon should have it available for reference at all times. Appropriate surgical conditions must also be maintained. The eyes are not occluded during the sinus procedure, as they are frequently examined and palpated during surgery. Adequate lighting is essential, and the endoscopes must be clean and functioning properly to achieve appropriate illumination of the intranasal surgical field. If the surgeon is uncomfortable with the endoscopic appearance of the nasal cavity or is confused by the anatomy, he or she should not hesitate to view the nasal cavity with a headlight if necessary in order to gain perspective. In addition, it is important to have excellent hemostasis, as operating in a bloody field is dangerous and should be avoided absolutely.

MAJOR COMPLICATIONS

For the purpose of this discussion, we will consider only the incidence, evaluation, and management of major complications of endoscopic sinus surgery. While synechia formation, lateralization of the middle turbinate, ostial occlusion, and other complications do occur, and are important in influencing the quality of the long-term outcome of the surgery, they are discussed in Chapter One. This chapter will therefore examine the more serious, immediate complications which can be encountered: orbital complications, intracranial complications, and massive hemorrhage.

Orbital Complications

Blindness

Clearly, the most feared complication of endoscopic sinus surgery is blindness. Blindness can occur through one of two mechanisms: direct injury to the optic nerve or compression of the optic nerve through retrobulbar hemorrhage. Optic nerve injury occurs most commonly in the posterior ethmoid cells[4] but can also occur through injury to the lateral wall of the sphenoid sinus. This posterior cell, often referred to as the *Onodi cell,* can extend laterally and/or superiorly to the sphenoid sinus, often confusing the surgeon as to its anatomic significance. In 12% of cases these cells are separated from the optic nerve by only a paper-like thinness of bone.[5] An examination of the preoperative CT scan is essential in identifying these superolateral posterior ethmoid cells.

The most common cause of temporary bleeding in the orbit is a retrobulbar hematoma.[6] This complication occurs primarily when there has been intraoperative injury to the lamina papyracea. In these cases, bleeding occurs within the orbit itself, causing an increase in intraocular pressure, thereby compromising the blood supply to the optic nerve and retina. When left untreated, orbital hematoma can cause significant visual loss, which can progress to permanent blindness in the affected eye.

The operating surgeon has several clues to the development of a retrobulbar hemorrhage. First, any penetration of the lamina papyracea must be viewed as a potentially problematic injury, and observation for further signs of a developing orbital bleed must be undertaken. Often the first sign to the operating surgeon of penetration of the lamina papyracea is the presentation of orbital fat in the lateral nasal wall. This fat has a more yellow color than the surrounding mucosa or polypoid tissue and will float in saline if placed in a specimen cup. In addition, palpation of the eye while observing intranasally will often transmit pressure to the orbital contents, causing movement of dehiscent fat or a fractured lamina papyracea as pressure is applied (Figure 12.1). Any orbital fat which is seen *must not be disturbed.* Do not attempt to trim or remove this fat. In addition, one must take special care in using powered sinus

surgical devices with exposed orbital fat, as this fat will be drawn into the cannula of the microdebrider and removed. A large amount of orbital fat can be quickly removed in this manner, so vigilance for and recognition of dehiscences in the lateral wall of the nose must be stressed. Silva and Stankiewicz[6] recommend admission of the patient for observation when fat is detected in anticipation of an orbital hematoma.

In addition to the visualization of orbital fat, other intraoperative signs of a significant orbital hemorrhage can often be detected. Periorbital ecchymosis, lid edema, chemosis, proptosis, and a tense eye are signs of a rapidly developing hematoma. In these cases, rapid intervention is necessary to prevent the development of permanent blindness in the eye due to ischemic injury. It is believed that 60 to 90 minutes is the maximal period of ischemia the retina and optic nerve can endure prior to the onset of irreversible damage.[7] However, depending on how quickly hematoma develops and the degree of elevated intraocular pressure, the amount of time available to reduce the pressure on the optic nerve may be as little as 15 to 30 minutes. It is important, therefore, that in these cases a strict protocol be followed to maximize the likelihood of preserving the patient's vision. The administration of mannitol, 1 to 2 g/kg intravenously, is begun immediately and given over a 30- to 60-minute period. Concurrent with the infusion of mannitol, orbital massage is begun immediately. Orbital massage redistributes the hematoma within the orbit, with subsequent

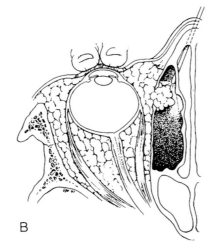

A   B

12.1. Technique of simultaneous eye palpation and intranasal endoscopic examination. **A:** Endoscope in place examining the lateral nasal wall and lamina papyracea. Note the hole in the lamina papyracea with mild fat exposure. **B:** Simultaneous eye palpation and endoscopic observation. If a hole in the lamina papyracea is apparent with periorbital or orbital fat exposed, early visualization of the defect is possible. (From Stankiewicz JA.[7] Reprinted with permission.)

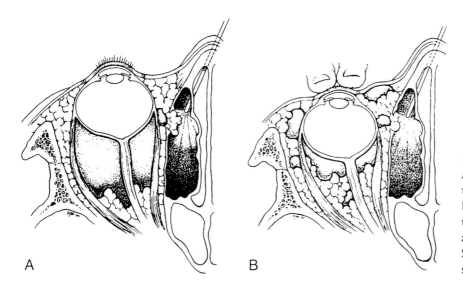

12.2. Technique of orbital massage. **A:** An orbital hematoma is noted after injury to the lamina papyracea and periorbita. **B:** Redistribution of the orbital hematoma and decreased intraocular pressure after orbital massage. (From Silva AB, Stankiewicz JA.[6] Reprinted with permission.)

reduction in intraocular pressure (Figure 12.2). Often with the use of these techniques alone, further problems can be averted. Ophthalmologic consultation should always be obtained in these circumstances for evaluation and follow-up of vision and intraocular pressure.

In situations in which the hematoma progresses and conservative measures fail to control the rise in intraocular pressure, lateral canthotomy with or without cantholysis is performed (Figure 12.3). This procedure is easily performed and will usually bring about a sufficient decrease in intraocular pressure to allow the process to resolve. In cases in which pressure remains high and vision is jeopardized, formal orbital decompression should be performed, either through an external Lynch approach or endoscopically. Bleeding can be controlled and the periorbita incised if necessary.

As always, when serious complications do occur, the patient and family must be advised of the events leading up to the complication, the treatment plan, and the prognosis.

Subcutaneous Emphysema

Subcutaneous emphysema arises from small breaks in the lamina papyracea in which air is forced into the orbit, resulting in puffiness, swelling, and crepitation of the eye. This event often occurs following vigorous sneezing, coughing, or anesthesia masking. While subcutaneous emphysema is usually benign and self-limited, the patient must be observed for signs of orbital hemorrhage, as the lamina papyracea has been disrupted.

Diplopia

Following sinus surgery, diplopia usually results from injury to the medial rectus muscle. This muscle lies just lateral to the lamina papyracea and can be injured if the lamina is damaged. While diplopia is usually transient, it can persist and can often be difficult to treat.[8] Referral to an ophthalmologist is always indicated when diplopia does not resolve spontaneously.

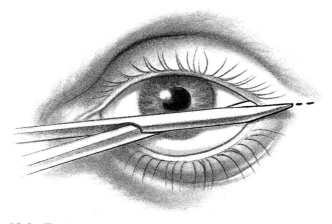

12.3. Technique of lateral canthotomy. (From Silver AB, Stankiewicz JA.[6] Reprinted with permission.)

Nasolacrimal Injuries

While symptomatic injuries to the nasolacrimal duct are rarely seen after endoscopic surgical procedures, occult injury can occur in up to 15% of patients.[9] The nasolacrimal duct is located just anterior to the natural ostium of the maxillary sinus (Figure 12.4) and can easily be injured in standard endoscopic procedures in which surgeons are instructed to complete their antrostomies anteriorly with a back-biting forceps. In powered dissection of the maxillary ostium, the antrostomy is created in a posteroinferior orientation, away from the location of the nasolacrimal duct. In most cases of injury to the duct, the epiphora will be transient. In cases of persistent tearing or recurrent dacryocystitis, a formal dacryocystorhinostomy may need to be completed.

Intracranial Complications

Intracranial injuries in endoscopic sinus surgery are noted in about 0.5% of cases.[10] The most common intracranial complication is cerebrospinal fluid (CSF) leak. Common areas of leakage are in the region just above the sphenoid ostium or sphenoidotomy openings[3] and in the anterior nasal cavity in the region of the lateral lamella of the cribriform plate. In addition, torquing of the middle turbinate can cause a skull base injury at its inser-

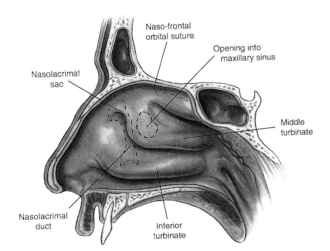

12.4. Relation of the nasolacrimal duct to the natural ostium of the maxillary sinus. (From Silva AB, Stankiewicz JA.[6] Reprinted with permission.)

tion superiorly.[11] Dura in this region is tightly adherent to the bone and can easily be torn through bony manipulation.

The first step in the repair of a CSF leak intraoperatively is its recognition. If the surgeon notes clear drainage with blood absent from the drainage area but surrounding the area (the *wash-out sign*) superiorly in the region of the sphenoethomoidal recess or the anterior nares, he or she should suspect the presence of a CSF leak. If it is recognized during the surgical procedure, repair of the bony dehiscence in the base of the skull can be completed as described below.

If the CSF leak is not identified intraoperatively, it can present following surgery as a slow but persistent clear rhinorrhea, often unilateral; it can also be perceived as posterior rhinorrhea into the pharynx. In these cases of immediate postoperative CSF rhinorrhea, initial management is conservative. The treatment protocol consists of strict bed rest for 1 to 2 weeks, avoidance of straining and nose blowing, and lumbar drainage if necessary.[12] While prophylactic antibiotic use has been controversial in cases of traumatic CSF rhinorrhea, in cases of CSF leakage during sinus surgery, bacterial contamination from the nasal and sinus mucosa is likely. In these cases, antibiotic prophylaxis with a broad-spectrum penicillin or cephalosporin is indicated. It is generally believed that a CSF leak which does not close spontaneously during this 1- to 2-week period is unlikely to close on its own and should be repaired.

In the repair of CSF leaks, autologous materials are preferred to artificial ones. Local flaps may be swung into position to close the defects, or free grafts of fascia can be harvested to be placed in the defect as tissue plugs. The use of lumbar drains at the time of repair of the CSF leak has been demonstrated not only to be ineffective, but also to increase patient morbidity in acute leaks.[13] Leaks present for more than 1 month dictate the use of lumbar drains as part of the operative protocol.

The defect is then visualized endoscopically using a 30° telescope. A small curet is used to freshen the wound edges, and 3 to 4 mm of dura is elevated to allow the fascial graft to slip under and close the wound. The graft can then be placed in position transnasally under the bony edges or positioned as an overlay graft. A small piece of Gelfilm is then placed external to the fascial graft. A square of non-adherent material such as Telfa is then placed, and this sandwich of packing is held in position with an expandable packing material such as Merocel. The packing is removed from the nose in about 10 days, but the crusting which remains superiorly is left in place until it extrudes spontaneously. When these extracranial approaches fail to control the CSF leak, a combined intra- and extracranial approach may be necessary to achieve a successful closure.

Hemorrhage

Significant hemorrhage following powered endoscopic sinus surgery is fortunately quite rare. In a large series of patients undergoing standard endoscopic procedures, the incidence of significant hemorrhage was only 0.19%.[10] Significant bleeding is known to be more common in patients with extensive disease and in patients who had undergone prior sinus procedures.[2] When significant bleeding occurs, it can do so from several locations. The majority of significant postoperative bleeds result from injury to one of the branches of the spheno-palatine artery. Often the location of this bleeding is in the lateral nasal wall near the insertion of the middle turbinate with the lateral wall or just below the sphenoid sinus. In addition, partial or complete resection of the middle turbinate can result in significant sphenopalatine bleeding. The use of the suction cautery in this area can provide excellent control of this type of bleeding, and if the physician's judgment dictates, nasal packing can be placed, to be removed postoperatively. It must be remembered that suction cautery must not be used within the sphenoid sinus or the orbit due to the risk of injury to critical structures.

Injury to the Internal Carotid Artery

Of more concern intraoperatively is hemorrhage due to injury of the internal carotid artery. The internal carotid lies in the lateral wall of the sphenoid sinus, creating a noticeable bulge in the lateral wall in 71% of cadaver specimens in one series.[14] In 4% of these specimens there was no bone separating the carotid from the sphenoid mucosa, and in 67% there was a bony covering of less than 1 mm. This incidence of bone less than 0.5 mm in thickness overlying the carotid artery has been reported to be as high as

88%.[15] Kennedy et al.[16] note that in endoscopic examination, 22% of internal carotid arteries are dehiscent in the lateral sphenoid wall.

Since the internal carotid is found in the lateral wall of the sphenoid sinus, it is important for the surgeon to enter the sphenoid sinus at its most medial portion when performing a sphenoidotomy. A thorough examination of the preoperative CT scan is essential to note whether any significant bulging of the artery into the sinus is present radiographically. If the surgeon stays near the midline, the sinus can be entered and examined endoscopically to evaluate the appearance of the sphenoid cavity and its lateral wall. Strict avoidance of any laterally based masses is critical. Only after the sinus has been examined endoscopically should the surgeon widen the ostium and perform any necessary dissection.

Iatrogenic injury to the internal carotid artery is a rare and often fatal complication of endoscopic sinus surgery. When intraoperative injury does occur, there may be immediate hemorrhage of variable severity, delayed hemorrhage, or the formation of a carotid-cavernous fistula. In addition, an intra-cavernous aneurysm of the carotid artery may result.[16] Most frequently, the injury to the artery will be apparent immediately. There will be a massive hemorrhage in these circumstances, which must be rapidly controlled with nasal packing and external compression of the ipsilateral carotid artery in the neck. Once the bleeding has been tamponaded sufficiently and the patient's vital signs stabilized, carotid angiography is performed to confirm the intraoperative injury and to determine its extent. If the initial bleed is now under satisfactory control, definitive therapy can be arranged. Angiographic balloon placement is often necessary in these patients to provide definitive control of the bleed, and arrangements must be made to transfer the patient to a facility where such treatment is available.

If the bleeding is controlled with packing, the patient is carefully monitored and the packing left in position for 1 week. Additional angiographic studies may be indicated to evaluate the thrombosis at the site of the injury. The packing can then be removed in the operating room setting and the patient observed for signs of further bleeding. Should bleeding recur, another pack is inserted and angiography with balloon occlusion is performed. The risks of occlusion are significant and must be reviewed thoroughly with the patient and family.

In cases of delayed hemorrhage, a similar protocol is followed. When the bleeding is controlled with nasal packing and when a significant injury to the internal carotid artery is anticipated, angiography is obtained immediately. Stabilization of the patient hemodynamically is critical, as is continuous monitoring in an intensive care setting.

It must be appreciated that the majority of intraoperative injuries to the internal carotid artery result in death or have serious neurologic sequelae if the patient survives. Attention to the radiographic anatomy on the CT scan preoperatively and good, careful surgical technique designed to prevent carotid injury is by far the more prudent course of action.

SUMMARY

This chapter has reviewed the most common major complications of endoscopic sinus surgery. Powered instrumentation can contribute to intracranial, vascular, or orbital injuries if the surgeon is not prepared, experienced, and prudent.

REFERENCES

1. Stankiewicz JA: Complications of endoscopic intranasal ethmoidectomy. *Laryngoscope* 97: 1270–1273, 1987.
2. Stankiewicz JA: Complications in endoscopic intranasal ethmoidectomy: An update. *Laryngoscope* 99:686–690, 1989.
3. Stankiewicz JA: Complications of endoscopic sinus surgery. *Otolaryngol Clin North Am* 22: 749–758, 1989.
4. Lawson W: The intranasal ethmoidectomy: evaluation and an assessment of the procedure. *Laryngoscope* 104:1–49, 1994.
5. Van Alyea OE: Ethmoid labyrinth. *Arch Otolaryngol* 29:881–902, 1938.
6. Silva AB, Stankiewicz JA: Perioperative and postoperative management of orbital complications in functional endoscopic sinus surgery. *Operative Tech Otolaryngol Head Neck Surg* 6:231–236, 1995.
7. Stankiewicz JA: Blindness and intranasal endoscopic ethmoidectomy: prevention and management. *Otolaryngol Head Neck Surg* 101:320–329, 1988.
8. Maniglia A, Chandler I, Goodwin W, et al: Rare complications following ethmoidectomies. A report of eleven cases. *Laryngoscope* 91:1239–1244, 1981.
9. Bolger WE, Parsons DS, Mair EA, et al: Lacrimal drainage system injury in functional endoscopic sinus surgery. *Arch Otolaryngol Head Neck Surg* 118:1179–1184, 1992.
10. May M, Levine HL, Mester SJ, et al: Complications of endoscopic sinus surgery: analysis of 2108 patients—incidence and prevention. *Laryngoscope* 104:1080–1084, 1994.
11. Rontal R, Rontal E: Studying whole-mounted sections of the paranasal sinuses to understand the complications of endoscopic sinus surgery. *Laryngoscope* 101:361–366, 1991.
12. Anand VK, Liberatore LA: Endoscopic cerebrospinal fluid repair. *Operative Tech Otolaryngol Head Neck Surg* 7:269–274, 1996.
13. Mattox D, Kennedy DW: Endoscopic management of cerebrospinal fluid leads and cephaloceles. *Laryngoscope* 100:857–860, 1990.
14. Renn WH, Rhoton AL: Microsurgical anatomy of the sellar region. *J Neurosurg* 43:288–298, 1975.
15. Fujii K, Chambers SM, Rhoton AL: Neurovascular relationships of the sphenoid sinus: a microsurgical study. *J Neurosurg* 50:31–39, 1979.
16. Kennedy DW, Zinreich SJ, Hassab MH: The internal carotid artery as it relates to endonasal sphenoethmoidectomy. *Am J Rhinol* 4:7–12, 1990.

13

Powered Endonasal Dacryocystorhinostomy

Michael Mercandetti, M.D., M.B.A., F.A.C.S
Joseph P. Mirante, M.D., M.B.A., F.A.C.S.

Dacryocystorhinostomy (DCR) is a technique to bypass an obstructed distal nasolacrimal system.[1] The obstruction is usually either in the distal nasolacrimal sac or in the nasolacrimal duct. Primary acquired obstruction of the nasolacrimal system is usually due to inflammation of an undetermined cause.[2] Patients with obstructed nasolacrimal systems often present with the signs and symptoms of epiphora and may suffer from acute and chronic dacryocystitis. Obstructions that are more proximal, such as at the internal punctum, the common canaliculus, or either of the canaliculi, are usually not correctable by a dacryocystorhinostomy. These cases usually require a conjunctivodacryocystorhinostomy (CDCR), whereby the proximal block is bypassed with a Pyrex-type tube.[3]

HISTORICAL PERSPECTIVE

Although high success rates with modern versions of the external dacryocystorhinostomy have been reported, many patients are concerned about the external scar, despite efforts to minimize it.[4] Other concerns include periorbital hemorrhage usually secondary to disruption of the angular vessels, epistaxis compounded by lack of visualization of the intranasal structures, and disruption of the tear pump mechanism, especially if the medial canthal tendon is affected. Other complications have included infection,[5] cerebrospinal fluid leaks,[6] and meningitis.[7] We will use the term *endonasal* to refer specifically to the use of the endoscope and *intranasal* for nonendoscopic approaches.

A major cause of failure in external, intranasal, endonasal, and laser dacryocystorhinostomies has been the closure of the ostium by scarring, granulation, and adhesions. Often the adhesions are between the ostium and the middle turbinate or the septum. Similarly the formation of synechiae and the lateralization of the middle turbinate have also been implicated as the causes of failure and recurrent disease in the endoscopic sinus surgery literature. The use of the microdebrider in powered endoscopic sinus surgery has been recognized as a promising technique in decreasing the incidence of many of these complications.

The first series examining the benefits of powered instrumentation in sinus surgery was presented by Krouse and Christmas in 1996.[8] Powered instrumentation was used exclusively in all aspects of the procedure, both soft tissue and bony dissection. In a group of 250 patients, the microdebrider was shown to afford faster healing, decreased bleeding, no synechial formation, and no middle turbinate lateralization. The authors postulate that the atraumatic dissection of the instrument through suction-dependent shearing of tissue causes less stripping of mucosa, leading to improved results. Use of the microdebrider for exposure through partial turbinate resection may provide for decreased ostial occlusion via less crusting, less scarring, less synechia formation, and less granulation tissue formation. We are continuing to investigate different techniques of mucosal resection, bony dissection, and creation of the ostium in primary and revision endoscopic dacryocystorhinostomy.

ANATOMY

In the adult, the lacrimal puncta are 0.3 mm to 0.5 mm.[9] The superior punctum is 5.0 mm, and the inferior punctum is 5.5 mm lateral to the medial canthal tendon. The vertical canaliculus is 2.0 mm long, and the horizontal canaliculus is 8.0 mm long. In approximately 90% of the population the inferior and superior canaliculi unite to form a common canaliculus 2 mm in length.[10] The entry of this common canaliculus is to the lateral portion of the nasolacrimal sac and is called the common internal punctum. Alternatively, the canaliculi can enter the sac separately. The nasolacrimal sac is 12–15 mm in length.[11] It is divided into a fundus, which is the area 4 mm superior to the medial canthal tendon, and a body which is below.[10] The nasolacrimal sac lies in the lacrimal fossa between the bony anterior and posterior lacrimal crests, adjacent and lateral to the lacrimal bone. The anterior lacrimal crest is formed by the thick bone of frontal process of the maxillary bone, and the posterior lacrimal crest is formed by the lacrimal bone. Superiorly, the sac lies just above the medial canthal tendon inferior to the cribriform plate, and inferiorly it extends to the inferior orbital rim where it connects with the nasolacrimal duct. The intraosseous part of the duct lies within the bony nasolacrimal canal for a distance of 12 mm, and the 5-mm meatal part of the duct lies lateral to the anterior and middle third of the inferior turbinate (Figure 13.1). The nasolacrimal canal is composed of the lacrimal and maxillary bones and the inferior nasal turbinate.

The lacrimal bone composes the anterior-superior part of the lateral wall of the nose. Rebeiz et al.,[12] in their cadaver study, determined that the mean diameter of the lacrimal bone was 1.13 cm. The distance from this bone to the bulla ethmoidalis was 0.49 cm, to the inferior turbinate was 0.91 cm, and to the anterior nasal spine was 5.11 cm.

The medial wall of the nasal cavity is formed by the cartilaginous and bony nasal septum. The perpendicular plate of the ethmoid and the vomer constitute the significant bony portion of the septum.

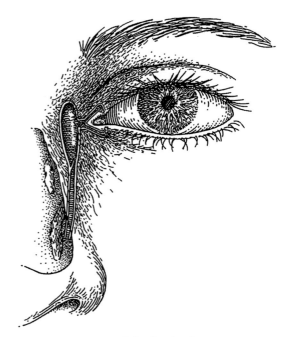

Figure 13.1. Diagram of the lacrimal system.

Anteriorly, the septum is formed by the quadrangular cartilage.

The lateral nasal wall is bounded by the maxillary and ethmoid sinuses and the orbit. The surgical anatomy is established by the mucosally covered conchae or turbinates, which are four horizontal projections from the lateral wall. Most critical to the nasolacrimal system are the inferior turbinate and the middle turbinate. The inferior turbinate arises from the lateral wall projecting horizontally to the choana posteriorly. It overlies the space of the inferior meatus. The inferior meatus houses the opening of the nasolacrimal duct. In a cadaveric study by Calhoun,[13] the distance from the anterior nasal sill to the nasolacrimal duct was 2.5 cm. The middle turbinate is a projection of the ethmoid bone. It overhangs and is parallel to the inferior turbinate. The associated space below the middle meatus is a key area in endoscopic turbinate. The associated space below the middle meatus is a key area in endoscopic nasal surgery. The medial wall of the nasolacrimal sac is generally located adjacent to the most anterior aspect of the middle meatus. The inferior edge of the sac is anterior and inferior to the insertion of the middle turbinate.

Botek and Goldberg[14] measured that the distance between the internal common punctum and the cribriform plate in five cadaver heads was 25.0 mm. Neuhaus and Baylis[6] created osteotomies in three cadaver heads with dimensions of 15 mm vertically and 18 mm horizontally. The distance from the superior aspect of the osteotomy to the cribriform plate averaged 5 mm with a range of 1 to 7 mm. Kurihashi and Yamashita[15] found in 28 Japanese cadaver heads that the mean distance between the floor of the anterior cranial fossa and the posterior lacrimal sac measured 8.3 mm with a range of 1.0 to 30.0 mm. In six of these heads, the distance was 3.0 mm or less. Botek and Goldberg[14] felt the larger distances to the anterior cranial fossa in their study compared to Kurihashi and Yamashita[15] were due to different reference points and ethnic anatomic differences.

SURGICAL TECHNIQUE

Powered endonasal dacryocystorhinostomy (PED) can be done under general anesthesia, or local anesthesia with concurrent intravenous sedation (MAC). Prior to bringing the patient to the operating room, the nose is sprayed with oxymetazoline 0.05% in order to initiate hemostasis. Xylocaine 1% with epinephrine 1:100,000 is then used for the regional block of the supratrochlear, infratrochlear, supraorbital, and infraorbital nerves. The nasal cavity in the area of the middle turbinate is anesthetized and vasoconstricted with cotton pledgets impregnated with 1:1,000 epinephrine. Local injection of 1% xylocaine with epinephrine 1:100,000 is given in the area of the lateral nasal wall. Injections are placed at the insertion of the middle turbinate, the anterior portion of the middle turbinate, and the mucosa anterior to the middle turbinate and middle meatus.[16] The injections are then given using a 25-gauge 1½-inch-long needle.

Attention is turned toward the eye where a protective plastic shield is placed to protect the globe (Figure 13.2). Topical ophthalmic tetracaine hydrochloride is administered prior to doing this to anesthetize the conjunctiva and cornea. The upper lid is retracted superiorly, while a lacrimal punctal dilator is directed perpendicular to the inferior punctum. The dilator is gently advanced into the punctum and the vertical canaliculus (Figure 13.3). Then, while the lower lid is placed on stretch laterally, the dilator is rotated to lie parallel with the lower lid margin. This stretching of the lower lid straightens the canaliculus, allowing for easier passage of the dila-

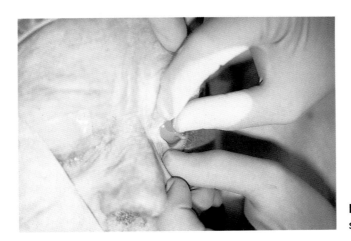

Figure 13.2. Insertion of the corneal shield.

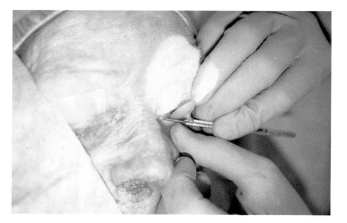

Figure 13.3. Cannulation and dilatation of the lacrimal punctum.

tor. The dilator is not twirled as this may create a false passage. The dilator is removed and a 0-0 (double zero) Bowman probe (0.69 mm diameter) is introduced into the punctum and canaliculus in a similar fashion. The probe is advanced approximately 8–10 mm until it abuts the thin medial wall of the nasolacrimal sac. The lacrimal bone can usually be felt through the sac, and this feeling is often described by the term "touching bone." If the passage is elsewhere, a more spongy feeling will be obtained and the sense of "touching bone" will be absent. In such an event, the probe can be directed slightly inferiorly while continuing to hold the lower lid on lateral stretch. If this fails, the probe should be removed and repassed. If the patient experiences discomfort while the dilator or probe is being passed in the canaliculus, 2–3 additional drops of tetracaine can be placed over the punctum, or a cotton pledget soaked in 4% xylocaine can be held over the punctum, after the dilator or probe is removed. After the 0-0 Bowman probe is passed, a 1-0 Bowman probe (0.89 mm diameter) is then passed, and this should enlarge the canalicular system adequately for the placement of the retinal light pipe or endoilluminator. A 20-gauge endoilluminator (Storz Instruments, St. Louis, Missouri), which produces cold light and is used intraocularly for retinal surgery, is introduced after the Bowman probe is removed (Figures 13.4 and 13.5).

Once inside the nasolacrimal sac, the endoilluminator is properly placed at a 45° angle to the horizontal plane at the medial canthus. At this juncture it can be taped into position. After placement of the endoilluminator, the gauze packing or cottonoids are removed from the nose and a 0° or 30° endoscope is used to visualize the lateral nasal wall just anterior to the middle turbinate. If necessary, the endoscopic light source can be dimmed to better visualize the light coming from the endoilluminator.

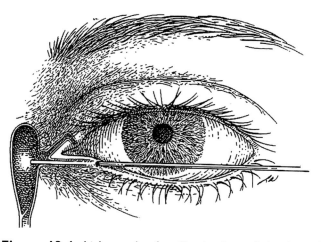

Figure 13.4. Light probe for illumination of the lateral nasal wall.

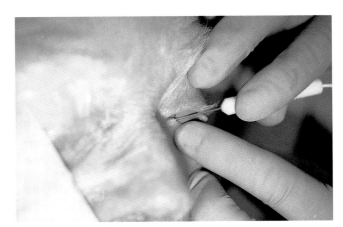

Figure 13.5. Insertion of the light probe into the punctum.

If the middle turbinate is closely opposed to this area and may block the ostium that will be created, the turbinate can be partially trimmed. This can be done with the microdebrider using a 3.0 serrated tip. Using the serrated edge, the mucosa of the anterior middle turbinate is roughened in order to obtain an edge for the instrument to grasp. Using a gentle rolling motion, the mucosa and underlying bone can be removed easily. The surgeon can then resect as much turbinate tissue as is felt necessary to provide

for a good postoperative meatus and to avoid stenosis. It is important in the use of powered instrumentation to have adequate suction pressure delivered to the handpiece in order to allow the tissue to be drawn into the inner cannula and sharply sheared and removed.

The point illuminated by the light carrier in the lateral nasal wall is the site in which the fenestration will be made into the lacrimal sac. The microdebrider is then placed (Figure 13.6) overlying this

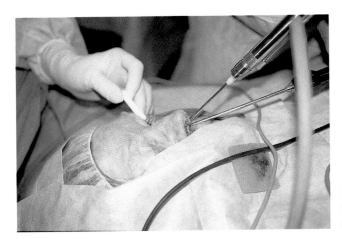

Figure 13.6. Insertion of the nasal endoscope and microdebrider for completion of endonasal dacryocystorhinostomy.

area of the lateral nasal wall, and the nasal mucosa is removed in a gentle fashion for at least 1.0 cm². As the mucosa is thinned and the bony cortex exposed, the surgeon will note an increase in intensity of the light. Depending on the age of the patient and the density of the bone, a curette can be used to create a small opening in the lacrimal bone overlying the endoilluminator. After the initial opening is made, the microdebrider is used in a rasping fashion to create an ostium with a diameter of at least 1.0 cm. The ostium is then enlarged with the powered device by removing the lacrimal wall, 10 mm in the superior to inferior direction and 8–10 mm in the anterior to posterior direction, with care being taken not to go too far superiorly or posteriorly, thereby remaining anterior to the uncinate process. Initially the surgeon may want to break the bone anterior to the endoilluminator, but it is not necessary to remove the frontal process of the maxilla which forms the anterior lacrimal crest. The endoilluminator usually rests in the inferoposterior aspect of the nasolacrimal sac. The nasolacrimal sac is usually seen after the bony ostium is made, and the endoilluminator can be removed at this point. However, it is usually left in and can be used to tent out the lacrimal sac. If the sac is scarred, a viscoelastic material can be injected via one of the canaliculi to dilate the sac.[17]

Once the ostium is formed, the sac can be incised with a sickle blade. The medial wall of the lacrimal sac is then removed with the microdebrider. The powered instrument is inserted through the opening into the sac created with the sickle knife, and with a circumferential rolling motion the sac is widened. The microdebrider can be used to combine the nasal and lacrimal sac mucosa. After the opening in the nasolacrimal sac is made, Guibor or Crawford-type silicone (silastic) lacrimal intubation probes are passed. The proximal ends of each metal probe are connected by an attached silastic tube. The probe is passed in the inferior punctum and canaliculus, as described for the Bowman probe (Figure 13.7). The distal end is passed through the opening in the nasolacrimal sac and the ostium into the nasal cavity from where it can be retrieved under direct visualization. The other probe is passed through the superior punctum and canaliculus which will most often have to be dilated. Dilation is done in a similar fashion as described for the lower punctum and canaliculus. The probe is retrieved from the nose and the metal probes are separated from the silastic tubing which is left in place as stents. Care must be taken to avoid pulling the tubes out of the nasolacrimal system at this point, and clamping the ends of the silastic tubing can assist in preventing this. The tubing is gently pulled to reduce the slack and tied with a

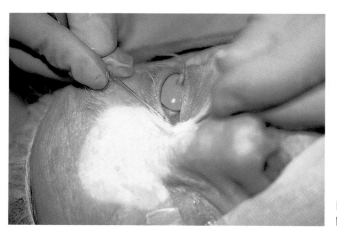

Figure 13.7. Placement of stent into the lacrimal punctum.

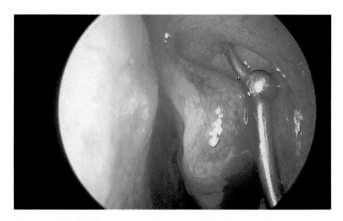

Figure 13.8. Patent window into the lacrimal sac postoperatively.

simple square knot. Care is taken to avoid placing tension on the tubing, thus making it too tight and causing it to erode or lacerate the puncti. Stents of differing materials can be placed over or into the ostium in addition to the tubes, in an effort to maintain the patency of the ostium.[18,19] We do not use additional stents.

Postoperative Care

The patient is placed on prophylactic antibiotics for 7–10 days. The patient should refrain from strenuous activity for the first 7 days. The patient uses a nasal decongestant spray for 72 hr and then uses nasal saline mist. Nasal steroids can also be used to decrease postoperative edema. The patient is seen at 1 week, at which time endoscopic inspection is carried out to assess the size of the ostium and remove excessive granulation tissue from around the ostium and stents, if needed. Follow-up continues at appropriate intervals to keep the ostium clear. The stents are removed at 2 months postoperatively (Figure 13.8).

CONCLUSION

The technique of intranasal dacryocystorhinostomy has undergone considerable refinement over the past several decades. Techniques have been de-

scribed using various approaches, including both laser and nonlaser methods. One issue which has continued to generate discussion has been the incidence of postoperative scarring and ostial stenosis, and the best method of reducing these complications.

The recent success of powered dissection of the paranasal sinuses and its demonstration to reduce significantly postoperative scarring and stenosis provide a promising framework for intranasal dacryocystorhinostomy as well. Early experience with the technique suggests that it can be performed easily and safely, and with minimal trauma to the normal mucosa of the turbinates and lateral nasal wall. Long-term data at this point do not exist, but as additional experience is gained with this approach, scientific assessment of these issues will be conducted.

REFERENCES

1. Conway ST: Evaluation and management of "functional" nasolacrimal blockage: results of a survey of the American Society of Ophthalmic Plastic and Reconstructive Surgery. *Ophthal Plast Reconstr Surg* 10:185–188, 1994.

2. Bartley GB: Acquired lacrimal drainage obstruction: an etiologic classification system, case reports and a review of the literature. Part 1. *Ophthal Plast Reconstr Surg* 8:237–242, 1992.

3. Jones LT: The cure of epiphora due to canalicular disorders, trauma and surgical failures on the lacrimal passages. *Trans Am Acad Ophthalmol Otolaryngol* 66:506, 1962.

4. Dortzbach R, Woog JJ: Small-incision techniques in ophthalmic plastic surgery. *Ophthalmic Surg* 21:615–622, 1990.

5. Walland MJ, Rose GE: Soft tissue infections after open lacrimal surgery. *Ophthalmology* 101:608–611, 1994.

6. Neuhaus RW, Baylis HI: Cerebrospinal fluid leakage after dacryocystorhinostomy. *Ophthalmology* 90:1091–1095, 1983.

7. Beiran I, Pikkel J, Gilboa M, et al: Meningitis as a complication of dacryocystorhinostomy. *Br J Ophthalmol* 78:417–418, 1994.

8. Krouse JH, Christmas DA: Powered instrumentation in functional endoscopic sinus surgery II: a

comparative study. *Ear Nose Throat J* 75:42–44, 1996.

9. Fein W, Daykhovsky L, Papaioannou T, et al: Endoscopy of the lacrimal outflow system. *Arch Ophthalmol* 110:1748, 1992.

10. Lemke BN: Anatomy of the ocular adnexa and orbit. In Della Rocca RC, Nesi FA, Lisman RD (eds): *Ophthalmic Plastic and Reconstructive Surgery,* Vol 1. St Louis, Mosby, 1987, pp 12–24.

11. McDonogh M, Meiring JH: Endoscopic transnasal dacryocystorhinostomy. *J Laryngol Otol* 103:585–587, 1989.

12. Rebeiz EE, Shapshay SM, Bowlds JH, et al: Anatomic guidelines for dacryocystorhinostomy. *Laryngoscope* 102:1181–1184, 1992.

13. Calhoun KH, Rotzler WH, Stiernberg CM: Surgical anatomy of the lateral nasal wall. *Otolar Head Neck Surg* 102:156–160, 1990.

14. Botek AA, Goldberg SH: Margins of safety in dacryocystorhinostomy. *Ophthalmic Surg* 24:320–322, 1993.

15. Kurihashi K, Yamashita A: Anatomical consideration for dacryocystorhinostomy. *Ophthalmologica* 203:1–7, 1991.

16. Kratky V, Hurwitz JJ, Ananthanarayan C, et al: Dacryocystorhinostomy in elderly patients: regional anesthesia without cocaine. *Can J Ophthalmol* 29:13–16, 1994.

17. Javate RM, Campomanes BS Jr, Co ND, et al: The endoscope and the radiofrequency unit in DCR surgery. *Ophthal Plast Reconstr Surg* 11:54–58, 1995.

18. Griffiths JD: Nasal catheter use in dacryocystorhinostomy. *Ophthalmic Plast Reconstr Surg* 7:177, 1991.

19. Woog JJ, Metson R, Puliafito CA: Holmium:YAG endonasal laser dacryocystorhinostomy. *Am J Ophthalmol* 116:1–10, 1993.

14

Powered Dissection in Otolaryngology: Future Directions

John H. Krouse, M.D., Ph.D., F.A.C.S.
Joseph P. Mirante, M.D., M.B.A., F.A.C.S.
Dewey A. Christmas, Jr., M.D.

It is clear that powered instrumentation in functional endoscopic sinus surgery has been a major contribution in the continuing refinement of surgical techniques in otolaryngology. From its early use as a device for removal of soft tissue in the nose, it has been modified and expanded to allow thorough dissection of all the paranasal sinuses with increased safety and precision. The pioneering efforts of a handful of otolaryngologists have permitted the successful adaptation of this technique from orthopedic surgery and oral and maxillofacial surgery to otolaryngology-head and neck surgery.

As with all new technologies, applications continue to be expanded as the users of that technology become familiar with its unique advantages. Increased comfort with a narrow range of indications leads to a gradual widening of the field until new indications and uses become developed, refined, and applied. Such is the case with powered instrumentation in otolaryngology. A variety of interesting applications has been implemented recently, and many of these uses will likely become part of the mainstream in otolaryngology as well as in other surgical disciplines. This chapter will discuss several of those interesting developments.

OFFICE-BASED POWERED DISSECTION OF THE SINUSES

Background

Several authors have described their experience with the use of powered microdebriders in the removal of polypoid disease of the nose in the office setting. The first surgeons to describe this technique were Hawke and McCombe,[1] who reported the successful use of a powered orthopedic shaver for office nasal polypectomy. They described that the procedure was quite easy to perform, had relatively little accompanying bleeding, and did not require the use of postoperative nasal packing.

Krouse and Christmas[2] also reported their experience with office nasal polypectomy. These authors described that the procedure could be done very easily with local anesthesia in the office, without the need for intravenous or oral sedation, and with comfort to the patient. Again, bleeding was minimal, and nasal packing was not necessary in their patients postoperatively.

Clearly there is sentiment within the medical community and supported by third-party payers to perform more surgical procedures in the office setting. A natural extension of the office-based technique for nasal polypectomy is the performance of noncomplicated ethmoid and maxillary surgery under local anesthesia in the office setting. In properly screened and selected patients, it is possible to perform limited ethmoidectomies and middle meatal maxillary antrostomies in the office without difficulty. Patient experience with this procedure can be acceptable, and can result in less complicated recovery periods and decreased cost to the patient.

Hemostasis and Anesthesia

The patient is seated comfortably in a chair with the head only slightly back during the entire procedure.

A chair which can be immediately placed supine is of great benefit for the procedure in the event of a vasovagal episode. As with all nasal and sinus surgery, attention to good hemostasis is critical in allowing a safe and precise procedure. The nose is first sprayed with a vasoconstricting agent such as ephedrine 3%, as well as with a topical anesthetic such as tetracaine 2%. After about 5 to 10 min has passed, cotton pledgets saturated with a combination of these two agents can be inserted into the nose, along the middle turbinates, and left in position for a few minutes. These pledgets can be used throughout the case for topical vasoconstriction in the event of minor oozing. After the pledgets are removed, injections of 1% xylocaine with 1:100,000 epinephrine can be made into the areas to be operated upon, including the middle turbinate edge, lateral nasal wall, and uncinate process. If polypoid disease exists in the nose as well, it can be injected directly and removed prior to the sinus surgery as described elsewhere in this text.[3]

Additional injections can be considered for field anesthesia depending on the extent of the surgery to be performed. An infraorbital nerve block can be of utility, and can be easily performed through the skin anteriorly at the level of the nerve. In addition, injection of the sphenopalatine ganglion through the foramen transorally can be performed for additional anesthesia more posteriorly, but the surgeon must be thoroughly familiar with this technique and its possible accompanying consequences.

Surgical Technique

Dissection of the sinuses is performed in a manner similar to that described by Christmas and Krouse for traditional hospital-based surgery.[4] The nasal cavity and lateral nasal wall are first examined with a 2.7-mm or 4.0-mm rigid nasal endoscope, and any anatomic abnormalities and pathologic findings are noted. It is very helpful to have the patient's CT scan available for reference during the surgical procedure.

It is initially important to identify the uncinate process, as this structure must first be removed in the completion of ethmoid and maxillary surgery. The uncinate process is tented out toward the surgeon with a ball probe or Lusk seeker, and its free

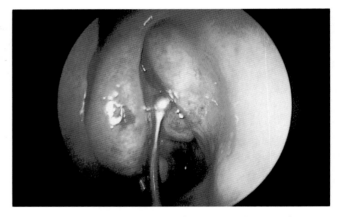

Figure 14.1. Ball probe identifying and palpating the uncinate process.

edge identified from superior to inferior (Figure 14.1). A small tear can then be made with the probe in order to allow an adequate grasping surface for the microdebrider. Utilizing a 4.0-mm serrated blade, the uncinate process is removed using a gentle rolling motion, allowing the tissue to be drawn into the rotating shaft without pressure (Figure 14.2). As the uncinate is removed, the bulla ethmoidalis is appreciated. It is crucial to remove the entire inferior remnant of the uncinate process, as residual tissue in this area can lateralize causing occlusion of the maxillary ostium, which is found immediately lateral to this portion of the uncinate.

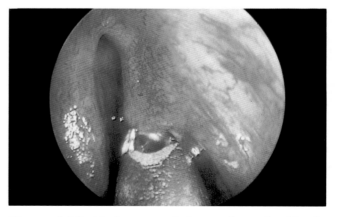

Figure 14.2. Uncinectomy being performed with the microdebrider.

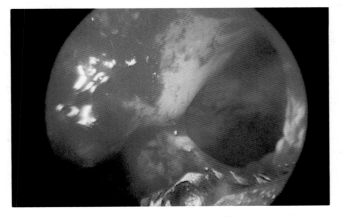

Figure 14.3. Enlargement of the maxillary antrostomy.

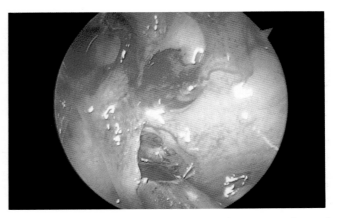

Figure 14.4. Microdebrider entering the anterior face of the bulla ethmoidalis.

At this point, the maxillary ostium can be visualized with either a straight or a 30° endoscope. If the ostium is patent and there is not significant disease of the maxillary antrum, no work needs to be done here. If the ostium is felt to be stenotic, or there is significant antral disease, the natural ostium can be widened in a posteroinferior direction. This procedure can be conducted by first making a small posteroinferior tear with the probe, and then utilizing the microdebrider to widen this area (Figure 14.3). The new convex maxillary sinus bits are especially useful for this procedure.

At this point, an ethmoid dissection can be performed. Again, as work proceeds posteriorly in the sinuses, it may be necessary to place additional topical pledgets for vasoconstriction and anesthesia, as well as performing additional injections of the local mixture. The microdebrider is then used to enter the bulla ethmoidalis anteriorly, punching through the anterior face, and then circumferentially widening this area with a gentle rolling motion of the device (Figure 14.4). Dissection can be continued through the basal lamella if necessary to approach posterior ethmoid disease. This circumferential rolling technique is used as the surgeon continues the dissection into the posterior ethmoid system.

At the conclusion of the dissection, rolled Gelfilm stents can be placed into the middle meatus to encourage healing. Care must be taken in placing these stents so as not to occlude the maxillary ostium. Nasal packing is not necessary in the majority of cases. Patients can then be observed for a few moments, and discharged home when ready.

Limitations

Obviously patient selection is paramount in the performance of sinus surgery in the office setting under local anesthesia. Children would not be good candidates for this technique, as they would be unable to cooperate. Consideration of this technique might be given to adolescents 15 or 16 years of age. In addition, patients who are anxious or apprehensive about surgery being performed awake in an office setting would also not be appropriate candidates.

Patients who have undergone prior surgery with some loss of landmarks also should not have this operation in an office setting. In these patients unexpected findings might be encountered, and the surgeon would be happier to be in a more controlled setting in this event. Extensive disease, or disease in the frontal or sphenoid sinuses might also be a relative contraindication to the use of the office technique at this time.

Finally, patients with significant concurrent medical problems would not be appropriate candidates for office surgery of this sort. Anyone with significant pulmonary or cardiac disease should be operated on in a more controlled setting with appropriate physiologic monitoring throughout the case.

Patients with a history of abnormal bleeding with surgery also should be approached in a more controlled surgical facility rather than in the office. The prudent use of the surgeon's judgment for this technique is the best guide in the appropriate selection of patients.

ENDOSCOPIC LIPODEBRIDEMENT

Background

Liposuction as a technique became popular in the late 1970s as a method for removing excessive adipose tissue and sculpturing the patient contour in cosmetic surgery.[5] The earliest reports of the procedure were from France in the 1920s.[6] These techniques have generally involved an avulsion technique in which force generated by the surgeon is used to displace the tissue and the suction used to remove it from the body. The cannulas and devices which have been developed for the performance of various liposuction methods have undergone very little modification over the past two decades.

Surgeons have been concerned about the precision of many of the original techniques in liposuction, motivating them to develop alternate strategies. Modifications have focused on a variety of factors including alterations in the shape and design of the cannula,[7,8] and on adjustments in the power and pressure of the vacuum.[9] While many of these techniques have refined the liposuction procedure, surgeons have continued to investigate methods to improve cosmetic results.

The first discussion of the use of powered dissection in the removal of subcutaneous adipose tissue was published by Gross and his colleagues in 1995.[10] They reported the use of the microdebrider in three cadaver specimens and two patients in which an open incision was made and the device used blindly to remove tissue from the subdermal fat plane. They reported in this limited series that ecchymosis seemed to be decreased when compared with usual techniques. In a follow-up study, Becker, Gross, and colleagues performed cosmetic facial surgery with the use of a microdebrider technique, coining the term "liposhaving" to describe this procedure.[11] The authors noted that the liposhaver was

used "successfully" in all cases, with symmetric contouring results and without dimpling of skin. There were no cases of facial nerve injury, no increased bleeding, and no hematoma formation in the immediate postoperative period. They feel that it may be a more safe and gentle technique in that suction pressures are lower than those used with traditional liposuction techniques. Again, the procedure was performed blindly.

Cosmetic liposuction as described above has been performed without direct visualization of the tissue planes during the surgical resection. One issue which may be pertinent is whether the use of a microdebrider device would increase the risk of injury to vital structures such as nerves, vessels, or muscular tissue. This question is raised by Gross et al. in their 1995 paper.[10] A similar question is raised by Hallock in the suction extraction of lipomas,[12] who notes that visualization of the adipose deposits aided in complete extraction of this material. Interest in endoscopic examination of the subdermal fat pad in suction lipectomy dates back to 1984.[13] In principle, an endoscopically guided approach to facial liposuction with a powered microdebrider would offer the precision and safety of the powered technology with the security of direct visualization of the operative field. In addition, endoscopic surgery can be performed through very small incisions, leaving much less postoperative scarring, a critical issue in cosmetic surgery.

Surgical Technique

The approach to endoscopic liposuction utilizing this technique is referred to as *endoscopic lipodebridement*. While this procedure can be performed in any fat plane of the body, for the present discussion we will concentrate on the head and neck. The procedure can be performed under either local or general anesthesia. After sterilely preparing and draping the surgical field (Figure 14.5), the site is infiltrated with 1% xylocaine with 1:100,000 epinephrine (Figure 14.6). Small incisions are then made overlying the fat to be excised (Figure 14.7), and a plane is elevated deep to the hair follicles of the skin under direct visualization with the endoscope (Figures 14.8 and 14.9). The fat pad is directly seen, and the microdebrider bit is inserted through

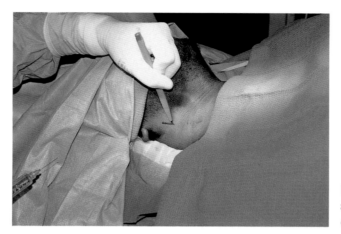

Figure 14.5. Neck prepared and draped and incision outlined for endoscopic lipodebridement.

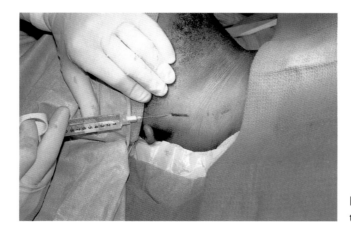

Figure 14.6. Infiltration of local anesthetic agent into incision site.

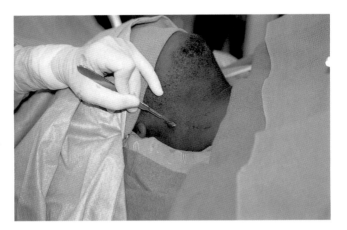

Figure 14.7. Incision being made into lateral neck for insertion of instruments.

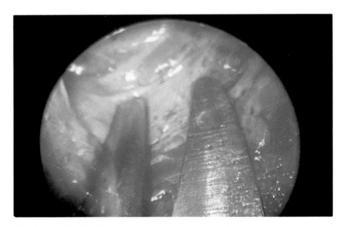

Figure 14.8. Endoscopic view of plane being created superficial to the cervical fat pad.

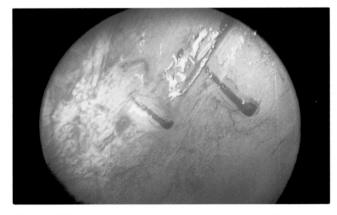

Figure 14.9. Hair follicles visualized endoscopically in the deep dermis.

the same incision (Figure 14.10). Any blood vessels or nerves can be noted and dissection can be performed so as to avoid any injury to these structures (Figure 14.11).

For dissection of the cervical fat pad, larger bits are more efficient in the removal of tissue than are bits of smaller dimension. Currently the limiting factor for many suppliers is the inner diameter of

the handpiece, which is in the range of 4.0 mm. One supplier, however, does manufacture a soft tissue shaver for head and neck use which accepts a 5.5-mm cannula, and would therefore have some advantages in the removal of cervical fat. In other sites of the head and neck, such as in the nasolabial fold area, a cannula of 3.0 mm would be more precise and appropriate. Smooth edged blades are suffi-

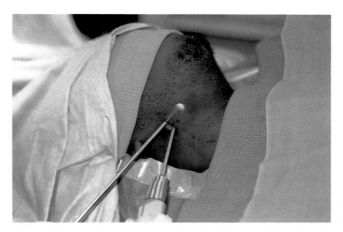

Figure 14.10. Insertion of the endoscope and microdebrider into the same neck incision.

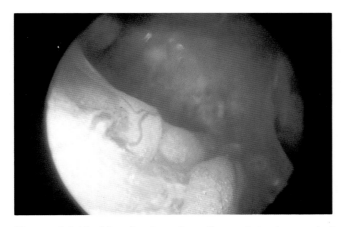

Figure 14.11. Visualization of small vessels in the cervical fat pad.

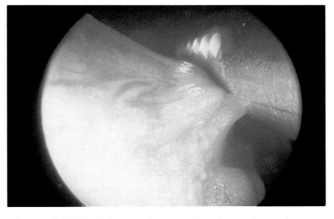

Figure 14.12. Adipose tissue being drawn into the cannula of the microdebrider and sheared free.

cient for the removal of adipose tissue, and avoid some of the secondary trauma which might be appreciated with serrated blades in this area.

At this point the device is actuated. Standard suction pressures are utilized as noted in sinus surgery, in the range of 170 to 180 mm Hg. A specialized liposuction vacuum device is not necessary as would be used in standard liposuction. The microdebrider is used in the oscillating mode to decrease blockage of the device. The surgeon directly visualizes the operative field at all times, and fat is drawn into the open port of the cannula by the suction pressure applied (Figure 14.12). Any vessels or nerves can be easily seen in this manner, and can be protected. The surgeon can directly gauge the amount of fat to be removed, deciding to

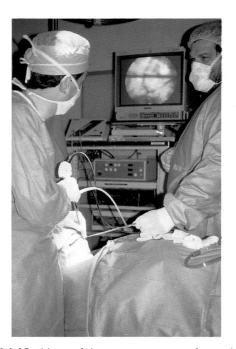

Figure 14.13. View of the operative setup for endoscopic lipodebridement.

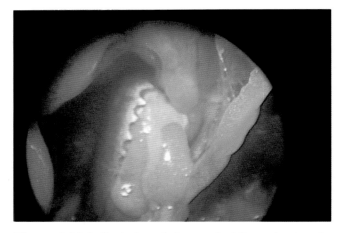

Figure 14.14. Sculpting of the cervical fat pad using the microdebrider.

remove greater or lesser amounts to achieve the desired contour (Figures 14.13 and 14.14). Once the fat pad has been sculpted to the amount desired, the instruments are withdrawn. At this point the incisions are closed using fine nylon suture material. Bulky dressings are applied as appropriate to limit postoperative bruising.

Observations

The impressions of surgeons who have utilized a powered approach to liposuction have been uniformly positive. Becker and colleagues reported decreased postoperative bruising and good healing in all patients. In their paper, however, they did report that visualization of the operative field increased precision and preserved soft tissues other than fat. They in fact preferred an open approach because of the precision it offered and the nature of their postoperative results.

A benefit of the endoscopic lipodebridement approach, then, is that it allows this direct visualization of tissue without the need for long open incisions. The precision of the dissection can be maintained through tiny incisions through which endoscopes can be passed and the tissue planes directly observed. Surgery, therefore, can be carried out precisely and safely under the direct visual guidance of the operating surgeon. It is this advantage which makes endoscopic lipodebridement the preferred method for sculpting of the fat pads of the head and neck.

While long-term research data have not yet been collected, the theoretical advantages of this technique are clear. Additional study is necessary in this area in order to more precisely delineate the parameters of this type of surgical procedure, and to develop a body of scientific knowledge which will demonstrate its safety and efficacy.

REFERENCES

1. Hawke WM, McCombe AW: How I do it: nasal polypectomy with an arthroscopic bone shaver: the Stryker "Hummer." *J Otolaryngol* 24:57–59, 1995.
2. Krouse JH, Christmas DA: Powered nasal polypectomy in the office setting. *Ear Nose Throat J* 75:608–610, 1996.

3. Mirante JP, Krouse JH: Powered nasal polypectomy. In Krouse JH, Christmas DA (eds): *Powered Endoscopic Sinus Surgery.* Baltimore, Williams & Wilkins, 1997.

4. Christmas DA, Krouse JH: Powered instrumentation in functional endoscopic sinus surgery I: surgical technique. *Ear Nose Throat J* 75:33–40, 1996.

5. Grazer FM: Suction-assisted lipectomy, suction lipectomy, lipolysis, and lipexeresis. *Plast Reconstr Surg* 72:620–623, 1983.

6. Caver C: The unpublished history of liposuction. Presentation at the Fourth Annual Scientific Meeting of the American Society of Liposuction Surgery, Los Angeles, January 1985.

7. Felman G: Felman double-liposuction cannula. *Aesthetic Plast Surg* 17:199–203, 1993.

8. Becker HA: A new suction cannula. *Ann Plast Surg* 25:154–158, 1990.

9. Lewis CM: Comparison of the syringe pump and aspiration methods of lipoplasty. *Aesthetic Plast Surg* 15:203–208, 1991.

10. Gross CW, Becker DG, Lindsey WH, et al: The soft-tissue shaving procedure for removal of adipose tissue. *Arch Otolaryngol Head Neck Surg* 121:1117– 1120, 1995.

11. Becker DG, Weinberger MS, Miller PJ, et al: The liposhaver in facial plastic surgery. *Arch Otolaryngol Head Neck Surg* 122:1161–1166, 1996.

12. Hallock GG: Endoscope-assisted suction extraction of lipomas. *Ann Plast Surg* 34:32–34, 1995.

13. Teimourian B, Kroll S: Subcutaneous endoscopy in suction lipectomy. *Plast Reconstr Surg* 74:708–711, 1984.

Index